KEEPING FACE

a Plastic Surgeon's Guide to Preserving and Improving Nature's Gifts

by

Robert L. Cucin, M.D.

Library of Congress Catalog Card No. 82-061104
ISBN: 0-9608304-2-1

FIRST EDITION

Table of Contents

PREFACE—FACING OURSELVES 7

PART I—FACESAVING 13

Above it all, the skin is the largest organ of the body; it is the fabric for the surgeon's craft. But its condition depends on *you!*

A. MAINTENANCE OF A YOUTHFUL AND BLEMISH-FREE COMPLEXION 13

1. Cleansing, Toning and Clarifying 15
2. Protecting and Moisturizing 21
3. Diet, Exercise and a Stable Weight 25
4. The System and Its Variations 31

B. SKIN SMOOTHING—IMPROVING DAMAGED SKIN 35

5. Face Masks and Facials 37
6. Removing Blemishes 39
7. Eradicating Acne Scars 43
8. Rejuvenating the Skin 47

C. SKINSHAPING—TAKING UP THE EXCESS 51

9. Eyelid Lifts 53
10. Face and Necklifts 63
11. Raising Sagging Brows 75
12. Lipshaping 83

PART II—FACEMAKING 87

Getting beneath the surface, the surgeon can change the scaffolding upon which the skin is draped and so sculpt faces to order.

A. FAT CONTOURING 87

13. Eliminating Eyelid Bags 89
14. Removal of Under-the-Chin Fat 97
15. Altering Puffy Cheeks 103

B. REARRANGING FACIAL MUSCLES 107

16. Alleviating Eyelid Festoons and Crow's Feet 109
17. Improving Jowls and Turkey Gobblers 115
18. Softening Frowns and Scowls 121

C. SOLID TISSUE SCULPTING 127

19. Enlarging the Eye 129
20. Treating Receded Chins and Flat Faces 135
21. The High Fashion Look through Cheek Implants 145
22. A Nose Sculpted for Your Face 153
23. Prominent Ears Placed into Perspective 175

AFTERWORD—FACING THE FUTURE 183

Preface
Facing Ourselves

FACING MYSELF

I must admit that I never wanted to be a "Doctor" in the traditional sense—one daily preoccupied with illness. I entered medicine knowing that my niche was to be in plastic surgery. However, I felt it was necessary to obtain full training and board certification in general surgery as well, to deserve the title of Doctor by first having to deal with life and death surgical decisions. Never-the-less, I'm quite happy that I no longer have to tell women that their breasts must be removed for cancer or men that they will never go to the bathroom normally again because of the treatment required for their rectal cancer. A patient is made much happier when his or her appearance is improved than when "cured" of cancer by drastic measures.

Since my teen years, I yearned to be a plastic surgeon. It seemed a wonderful skill and gift to be able to share with people. My dream began after an encounter with a young boy who had been born with severe facial deformities—one side of his face totally misshapen with a missing eye and tiny eye socket, an absent jaw, and other defects. He at first appeared to be barely human and could not pass publicly without conspicuous stares. But over the next decade, I kept in touch as he underwent multiple plastic surgical procedures. The results were absolutely astounding! After each procedure, he came to look more and more like a normal person. Even more astonishing were the changes in his personality along the way. From an obnoxious, insecure, abrasive individual, he became a more well-adapted, confident person. Today, he is a successful businessman—not wildly handsome, but not carrying the visual stigmata of a congenital defect. He is now able to mingle socially, date, and pass as normal.

What a gift of quality of life has been given to this young man by the many plastic surgeons who had labored over him! How different his life might have been—perhaps even hidden in the back ward of an institution had he not been availed of "the kindest cut"—the scalpel of the plastic surgeon. I came to realize that gross defects were not the only ones that can impair a person's quality of life. Even seemingly small defects—such as a hooked nose—can be monumental to some individuals and inhibit their full participation in the world around them.

The second factor in my decision to be a plastic surgeon arose as I discovered women. Frankly, women fascinate me, and I delight in their company. A woman who is confident about her appearance radiates such a glow, an invitation to get to know her. How often have I seen women experiencing the ravages of aging—the sagging jowls, the drooping eyes, the wrinkles—still handsome women but obviously dismayed with the changes of time. How dreadful that such women may shrink from the exciting experiences life has yet to offer, considering themselves "too old". I believe that women are never "too old" to be entrancing.

My last reason for entering the field was that, being meticulous about my own appearance, it is very easy to emphathize with any patient—man or woman—who wants to look as well as possible. Some people would agree with the "right" of the man with birth defects to have plastic surgery, but scorn those who seek "cosmetic" surgery. I strongly disagree! What good is it to tell the woman whose face is aging that our culture is "youth oriented" and that she should not be dismayed by her changing image in the mirror? Our society *is* what it is, and she is realistically disturbed. She wants not to be a raving beauty, not to be something she never was, but simply to have the hands of time turned back and slowed down a bit. She wants to continue to look *her best*. It is for such *women—and men and children*—who want to look *their best*, that plastic surgery can provide an invaluable service.

Upon entering the field, I soon learned the origin of the word doctor was from the Latin verb *docere*, meaning *teacher*. This is a responsibility I take quite seriously and is one of the reasons for which I wrote this book. I consider it essential that my patients be fully informed. Obviously, the topic of plastic surgery is very important to me. If you have ever considered having plastic surgery or someone you love has considered it—this book is essential reading. Plastic surgery has been around for a long time—since 600 B.C., according to ancient records. But many techniques have changed dramatically in the last decade, and new procedures have become available. Where can a person considering plastic surgery get the latest solid information on what's involved? Magazine articles must be necessarily brief, and some of the books published in past years gave an overly glamourized view of plastic surgery.

Plastic surgery is very different from the other medical subspecialties, How is it different? Well, when people go to a doctor, they usually are sick and do not know what is wrong with them. The doctor tells them what is wrong and what he will do about it. Then the patient "follows doctor's orders". In the practice of plastic surgery, the roles are almost totally reversed. Typically, the patient comes to the plastic surgeon *knowing* what he or she considers to be wrong. The patient tells the physician what he or she wants done about it. The plastic surgeon then advises the patient whether or not it *can* be done, how easily, and if it will indeed give the desired result. If the answers to these questions are favorable, the patient then gets precisely what was sought. *Plastic surgery is the ultimate in consumer-oriented medicine.*

Yet, even in this specialty, designed to meet the needs of the consumer/patient, I have seen less than happy results—patients with inappropriate expectations, patients who failed to communicate their real desires to the physician, physicians who failed to fully explain what could or could not be done or what could go wrong—as well as people who never sought their "visual dream" because they thought it could not be achieved or because they thought there was "something wrong" with wanting it. I believe that all of us—man, woman or child—have a right to look our best according to our own personal standards and values of what "best" is . . . every day of our lives. However, I consider it extremely important—vital—that people embark on a plastic surgical experience *fully informed*—from how they should prepare for surgery, to what to expect during surgery, to how they will look and feel in the weeks, months and years after surgery. It is the purpose of this book to bridge the information gap that exists today—between the dreams of millions of people and the reality of what plastic surgery can offer.

While questioning patients about the skin care they practiced before during and after treatment of their problems, I very quickly saw a need for guidance on the subject—both to *prolong* and *enhance* the results of my surgical endeavors and prophylactically to *postpone* or even *prevent* the need for future surgical intervention. A good portion of the questions addressed to me by my patients was about skin care. Based upon current research, my observation of the greater or lesser effectiveness of different marketed products upon my patients, and in response to their particular problems, I developed a selection of skin treatments. This selection, after being repetitively refined and reformulated with extensive clinical experience, grew into a full skin treatment line and skin care system which my patients began recommending to their families and friends. Since I have no direct contact with many of these persons now employing the line, I have no way of reaching them *except* through this book.

FACING YOURSELF

We all have self-images, which in some cases may be quite accurate, but, in others may depart from reality rather remarkably. They may be based on self-images formed in childhood or early adulthood that have not been modified in years, while pounds have accumulated and wrinkles have multiplied.

To obtain full benefit from this book, it would be well, in the privacy of your home, to sit down comfortably facing a mirror and remove all traces of make-up. In good lighting, you can now examine yourself carefully and make notes as to what you see so that you can pay particular attention to the portions of the book that most apply to you.

First, take note of your skin itself. Does it appear oily and shiny? Are your pores large? Are there troublesome eruptions of blemishes in any area of your face or blocked pores and blackheads? Does your skin appear dry, scaly or sore looking?

Is your skin mottled or leathery—old before its time? Are there any broken capillaries or spiders? Do you have acne, chicken pox or other scars, any growths, or discolorations? Are there numerous crow's feet radiating from the corners of your eyes? Are there fine lines radiating from your lips? Are your lips too full or thin?

Do your eyes suggest you were up all night because of lower eyelid bags or dark rings beneath them? Is there extra skin above the upper lid? Do your eyes appear too small? Has your brow slipped downwards somewhat? Do scowl lines give you an angry look? Do you have forehead wrinkles? Do deep laugh lines or jowls bracket your mouth and jaw? Do you have a clean neckline or an under-the-chin fat deposit with a "double chin"?

Next, examine the proportions of your face. Does your face appear round or flat? Do you have a low forehead or a forehead too high with a receding hairline? Are your cheekbones well-pronounced or barely visible? Are your cheeks puffy? Does your face show the presence of a few extra pounds? Does your chin recede somewhat or does your jaw protrude too far forward?

Does your nose give a fairly straight profile or is it too bobbed or humped? Does the tip of your nose droop down too far? Is the nasal bridge so wide that it detracts from your eyes? Is your nose so long that your upper lip disappears beneath it when you smile?

Are your ears sticking out too far or have your earlobes grown out of proportion to the rest of your ear?

You are free to look, examine and objectively record your findings. If there is anything you may notice, it is readily *treatable*; some of it simply; some of it with greater difficulty—but all of it is treatable. If you like everything you see, terrific! This book *still* has something most important to offer you—it will help you to discover how to *protect* and *preserve what Nature has given you.*

Because of my desire to present a "no nonsense", current and accurate guide to what plastic surgery can offer and my observed need for similar advice on the subject of skin care, I organized this book into two parts—the first, *Facesaving*, begins with skin care and the preservation of what Nature has given us. It then discusses the non-surgical and surgical skin treatments directed at correcting nature's imperfections and the damage we ourselves may have caused.

The second section of the book, *Facemaking*, goes beneath the surface and discusses plastic surgical procedures directed at the deeper problems of aging and less-than-perfect inherited and acquired facial aesthetics. So *make your notes and read on . . .*

* * *

PART I
FACESAVING

A. Maintenance of a Youthful and Blemish-Free Complexion

CHAPTER 1

Cleansing, Toning and Clarifying

The skin constitutes the largest organ of the body; we have between one and two square yards of it and it is the envelope holding the human contents we know of as you and me. With the exception of the blind, cave-dwellers, and the extremely myopic, the impression it makes upon others is inescapable. As a plastic surgeon, I can do wonders with the skin—but—*its condition depends on you! The treatment of your skin today determines its condition tomorrow.*

Like any other organ of the body, the skin contains cells which require nutriments and excrete wastes. However, unlike any of the other organs, the skin is specialized as an interface with the outside world; it has adapted to protect the body from the environment. The small blood vessels deliver oxygen and glucose to the skin and remove its wastes. The cells rapidly renew themselves as the old ones are sloughed away. You can see the buildup of dead cells in calluses. That the skin cells readily come away can be seen in our ability to remove ink from the hands by friction alone.

The external location of the skin is the source of several distinct problems in the maintenance of its health; namely, it is exposed to damaging sun and ultraviolet light, wind, salt, pollutants, irritants, allergenic compounds, dirt, detergent residues in clothing, friction and chafing, perfumes, colognes, make-ups, shaving creams, depilatories, anti-perspirants, hair sprays and hair grooming aids, and drying conditions. With all these exposures, it is indeed a wonder the skin does as well as it usually does! Fortunately, Nature has specialized it very cleverly so that it usually stands up to these multiple onslaughts quite effectively. However, many of the chemical and synthetic molecules and compounds to which it is now exposed were not among those which Nature "anticipated". For example, Nature never expected a full coat of make-up!

Routine "dirt" from the soil could be removed in Nature quite easily with water from a flowing stream or the saliva from a licking tongue. However, most people today never get any closer to the soil than their potted plants; therefore, the cleansing agents they use must be able to deal with modern problems and contaminations. These more capable cleansing agents will all remove certain intrinsic moisturizers and protectants from the skin that should be replaced in the process of toning and moisturizing. Ideally, the skin care system will employ a cleansing agent that leaves no residue on the skin to block its pores or cause allergic reactions (either by itself or by reaction with the sun) and will "strip" the skin only minimally while being able to deal effectively with make-ups and modern pollutants.

Soaps are salts of fatty acids that leave stearate residues on the skin which are drying and can be irritating, particularly if scented. Their alkalinity encourages pollutants to "stick" to the skin making the face feel "dirty" again. If a soap is to be employed, the least objectionable is the glycerine and rosewater variety because it is less drying and irritating, and leaves the least objectionable residue. It does not "strip" the skin quite as badly as the other soaps. However, in preference to soaps, I strongly prefer and recommend cleansing agents that do not dry the skin, strip minimally, and do not leave objectionable residues. These agents are formulated into solution as either liquids or lotions. Of these two forms, I prefer the lotions for their ease and economy of application.

Since, as we have discussed, any cleansing agent will remove some of the skin's intrinsic protecting and moisturizing factors, these must be replaced following cleansing. That brings us to toning and moisturizing. A toner should remove whatever minimal residue the cleanser leaves and tighten the skin so that pores and fine wrinkles are less visible. It does this by "plumping" up the cells. It should leave the face feeling clean, alive and fresh and with a healthy "glow". It restores the pH balance of the skin. The moisturizer which follows will replace whatever has been removed by the cleanser and protect the skin from all the damaging things to which it is exposed.

Cleansing lotions should be applied with warm water. Chemical reactions such as cleansing are promoted by heat; however, the water should *not* be so hot as to harm the skin. Mild sloughing is encouraged by applying the cleanser on a soft, gentle and clean washcloth. The washcloth should be changed daily and even more frequently if there are any active eruptions. Rough cleansing encourages scaling, cracking, broken blood vessels, and "spiders". I strongly dislike buffers and coarse grainy cleansers. I discourage their use—or perhaps I should say misuse—because the mechanical advantage of their roughened surfaces makes it too easy to do damage. The cleansing lotion, softened make-up, and removed dirt should then be washed off with cool water to close the pores.

In its relation to the outside world, the skin offers one convenience to us—direct access. We can make topical application of substances designed to keep it in good shape. Namely, we can apply moisturizers designed to retain water against the skin and chemicals designed to be absorbed by the skin for a desired effect. The moisturizer should replace all that is lost in the process of cleansing and provide an abundance of that required for maintaining the softness and *turgor* (cellular tone) of the skin. It should do this without causing allergy or blocking pores. Too "rich" an agent can possess both of these drawbacks. One with oily skin cannot use as "rich" a moisturizer as one with dry skin. The latter person not only can but *should* use a moisturizer formulated for that problem. Older and sun-damaged skin usually is less oily than younger skin that has been kept out of the sun.

The skin changes in oiliness throughout our lives. The sebaceous glands are more active during adolescence when the male and female hormones are actively secreted and during periods of emotional stress. The central face or "T zone" of the face is usually more oily than the rest of the face. We all really have "combination" skins—it is just a question of degree—*this is normal.* Many skin treatment lines have restricted the definition of "normal" so narrowly that we all are abnormal. This simply is *not* true.

Dealing with the periods of stress, adolescence, and emotional breakouts of troublesome eruptions brings us to the clarifying lotions. A clarifying lotion should be capable of unblocking the pores and preventing the transition from a blackhead to a pimple or pustule. It is not required all the time but *only* at these times. It, too, will remove certain natural protectants from the skin. These must, just as when removed by cleansers, be replaced in subsequent moisturizing. Obviously, under these conditions, the moisturizer applied afterwards should not be very "rich". Clarifying lotions can be formulated to cleanse at the same time; however, rather than formulating multipurpose mixes, I prefer simple lotions designed to accomplish one thing at a time and perform that task well. A cleanser should cleanse and a clarifying lotion should do just what its name implies!

Intrinsic in their nature and alcohol content, clarifying lotions will simultaneously tone and, when employed, can usually be substituted for the toning lotion. This should be so to maintain simplicity in the regimen and restrict it to only three steps. This simple *1-2-3 step system* of skin care is to *CLEANSE, TONE OR CLARIFY, AND MOISTURIZE.*

Both toning and clarifying lotions are best applied with cotton puffs which are discarded after use. These necessitate use of very little and provide convenience in application. Obviously hands should be washed before touching the face in any way. *Cleanliness will be best maintained if hands are kept away from the face.* Then it does not matter if strong agents are used to clean the hands or if they leave harsh residues. The skin of the hands is our major direct contact with the world; this obviously creates a separate set of problems for these highly specialized organs which are not the subject of this guide.

In the morning, men should apply the cleansing lotion in routine fashion but rinse it off with *warm* water before applying their shaving cream and shaving. Then, after rinsing off the shaving cream with *cool* water, they should follow through with steps 2 (toning or clarifying) and 3 (moisturizing). A good aftershave or "skin-bracer" aspires to be a toner; step 2 should replace the use of an aftershave. Some men will prefer the use of the clarifier as an "aftershave" because of the delightful tingling sensation it gives the skin. Since most men have oilier skin than their female counterparts, using the clarifier in the morning and the toner in the evening in step 2 generally works out quite well.

Having spoken about two variations of the regimen, namely, cleansing-*toning*-moisturizing or cleansing-*clarifying*-moisturizing—depending on whether the skin is initially clear or blemish-ridden—it is evident that normal care will be *toning* and that *clarifying* should be required only during periods of stress or for initially clearing up the skin. The difference will be the substitution of a clarifying agent for the toner in step 2 transiently to clear up the skin. This will probably be required from time to time—such as while traveling, during periods of emotional upheaval, and perhaps around menses.

All cleansers, toners, clarifiers, and moisturizers should be applied with a *gentle touch* and *in an upwards direction* as as to help the face retain its youthful character. The clock will tick on without us pushing the pendulum faster! Two washings should suffice to remove all but the most caked-on dirt and make-up.

A word must be said about the individual agents chosen. It was mentioned that they should be *compatible with one another* and designed *as a system* with the end result in mind—a clear skin. It is easiest and usually best to use the skin care products designed by one laboratory to obtain this goal rather than the hit-and-miss approach of trying a supermarket soap, a toner from a doctor, and one of the plethora of cosmetic company moisturizers. The likelihood of optimal results from a *potpourri* skin care regimen like this is poor and the probability of cross-reactions and allergy high.

Any new regimen will require a few days to two weeks to get used to and evaluate; however, in beginning a regimen, no severe eruptions should occur during the first few days. Occurrence of rashes or similar reactions in the past suggests allergy to one of the products contained within the line. If another product has caused a similar reaction, it is well to "play detective" and *check the labels* to see if the same ingredient is listed in both products. A doctor may be able to point out the ingredient(s) most suspect which should be avoided in the future. Skin tests are possible to confirm the suspicion but seldom are actually required.

The *1-2-3 regimen should be applied twice daily*; first in the morning and then in the evening. The moisturizer in each case, however, should not be the same but be formulated with a different purpose in mind. But more about that later . . . (Chapter II).

* * *

CHAPTER 2

Moisturizing and Protecting

As cells migrate from the deeper layers of the skin to more superficial locations, they become lifeless, keratinize and eventually flake off. The skin provides a barrier between the moist tissues beneath and the drying world without. It provides its own protective secretions to keep itself from drying out. In older, drier or sun-damaged skin these may not be sufficient. They usually are not sufficient in arid, sunny climates or with dry central air heating. These factors are also removed in cleansing. Because of this, it is necessary to supplement and replace the skin's own protection on a regular basis to maintain the best possible complexion. A moisturizer will *protect* the skin from drying, *hold water against the skin, replace* the natural skin protectants removed by cleansing, and *supplement* those deficient in quantity or quality.

The sebaceous glands of the skin secrete a complex lipid (fat) mantle designed to provide a moisture barrier. One of the principal ingredients of this lipid mantle is *squalene*. Since it's one of Nature's principal protectants, I recommend its inclusion in moisturizers since "Nature generally knows best." *Linoleic acid* is another fatty acid found in the skin and I advocate its inclusion for this same reason.

The use of collagen for high value skin care preparations was stimulated by the extensive medical investigations of the positive influence of collagen on wound healing, by investigations of the relations between age and alterations of collagen, as well as by the general use of collagen preparations in human medicine, especially in surgery. Collagen constitutes the structural protein used as the steel girders for the edifice of the body. It comprises about 83% of the skin and bone. Personally working with soluble collagen preparations in 1970, I developed a strong clinical impression that collagen had a positive influence upon the healing of *damaged* skin although our studies did not provide the clear-cut clinical proof we obtained with bony healing studies. Collagen absorbs many times its weight in water; therefore it is one of the most effective substances for holding water against the skin in addition to any direct effect it may have.

There are relatively few compounds that can cross the keratin barrier of the skin and enter cells. DMSO (dimethyl sulfoxide) is one; we once hoped it would be the "wonder carrier" for transporting desired substances across the keratin barrier of the skin. Unfortunately, it is not safe to use clinically as it can cause cataracts. From my own work and those of others in skin preservation, it has been shown that glycerin and the glycols freely enter the cells. They are wonderful humectants and the "work horses" of most moisturizers. They are usually combined with lanolin and sorbitol in most preparations to increase effectiveness.

Elastin and other insoluble molecules cannot cross the keratin barrier; besides being difficult to formulate they *add little* except expense to moisturizers. For these reasons, I recommend against their use.

The main action of *Vitamin A* (Retin A) is to restore normal keratinization in conditions in which it is disturbed. It enhances DNA synthesis in the germinative epithelium and increases the mitotic rate (the rate at which the cells renew themselves). It has been used for a number of skin disorders characterized by follicular plugging, abnormal keratinization, acne, psoriasis and senile (solar) keratoses. The risk of sensitization is small. For all these reasons, I recommend its inclusion in the moisturizers used.

Vitamin D has long been used in combination with Vitamin A in emollient ointments for providing soothing relief for abrasions, minor burns and chafing. It helps form the moisturizer's water-proof shield to protect against abnormal dryness while being an infrequent cause of reactions. *Vitamin B_5* (Pantothenic acid) has been shown to be a dietary requirement of most other mammals, but not in man. It is necessary for the formation of a vital enzyme (Co-enzyme A) in metabolism and has nice formulating properties for moisturizers. *Vitamin E* (alpha-tocopherol) has been shown to have favorable anti-inflammatory and anti-scarring effects and seems to warrant inclusion in spite of its slight sensitization possibility which can be minimized by the form selected.

The moisturizer chosen for step 3 should fulfill different requirements for day-time and night-time use. In the day time, when used under make-up and in public, the cream should "vanish" almost instantly without a visible trace. It must not cause difficulty in applying make-up or "transfer" of the make-up after application; it should not make the skin appear greasy or shiny. It must provide an invisible protection against drying and prevent pollutants and dirt from becoming deeply embedded. Since the sun is a principal cause of cellular aging, a protection against its ill effects is desired. *Mexenone* has been shown to be highly effective in this regard and is only rarely the cause of sensitivity reactions. I advocate the inclusion of it or a similar agent in the day-time moisturizer for these reasons.

The night-time moisturizer may be somewhat "richer" than that used in day-time since problems of make-up need not be considered. It does not have to "vanish" quite as rapidly but should have a continued effect throughout the night. It should not block the pores while having this favorable effect or it will cause as much damage as good. Obviously, no sunscreen is required or desired. Application of both night-time and day-time moisturizers should be in a *gentle, upwards direction* and *with clean hands.* A glycerine and rosewater soap or *preferably a soapless cleanser* are good for preliminary cleansing of the hands.

Eyelids constitute a separate consideration. Since the skin is so thin and delicate, it has virtually none of the protectants of the facial skin. However, eyelids frequently appear puffy if oily moisturizers are used upon them. I advocate use of a very pure, vanishing, relatively bland and oil-free moisturizer for the eyelids to help prevent crow's feet and crepey skin. Usually, application at night-time is all that is required. Eyelids should be handled *very gently* and *with clean hands.* Avoid getting the eyelid cream in the eyes; do this by applying it sparingly.

Bright sunlight such as on ski slopes and beaches represents a severe threat to the maintenance of a youthful skin. While there is no question of the immediate "cosmetic concealing effect" of a tan to cover blemishes, this apparently favorable effect is only transitory. *Each sunburn causes a small injury with definite, and probably irreversible, damage to the skin.* It destroys the collagen and elastin in the dermis. Sun abuse will cause a leathery, mottled and prematurely-aged skin prone to multiple growths and discolorations—*including malignancies.* Every plastic surgeon has a multitude of patients in his practice who come back, year after year, with fresh skin cancers for excision. It gets monotonous for both surgeon and patient. Unless you wish to be a member of this patient population—*protect your skin from the sun!*

Unless you have had either a chemical peel or dermabrasion, both of which make it more likely for you to burn and less easy for you to tan, or are very fair or a burn-no-tan redhead, direct sun exposure in moderate climates can be dealt with a moisturizer with SPF (sun protection factor) 6-9. This is light enough protection to still allow some tanning—but heavy enough to prevent burning and damage to most skins. If you fall into any of the previously mentioned categories or are in tropical climiates, SPF 12-15 is advisable. *PABA*, para-amino-benzoic acid, is the highly effective ingredient for protection against the damaging wavelengths of sunlight. There is a low incidence of allergic reactions to this compound, so it is advisable to do a small "patch test" on the inside of your elbow before applying to your face for the first time.

For all the reasons behind employing a moisturizer at all, it is especially important than one be employed in direct sun. Protection from salt, wind, and sun requires a good "moisture barrier". I could not agree more with the old proverb, "Only mad dogs and Englishmen go out in the midday sun!" If you like sports which place you in the sun—such as tennis, swimming, or golf—*protect your skin.* As for deliberate sun-bathing or "sun-baking", I cannot strongly enough emphasize how damaging and prematurely aging it is to the skin!

If sun damage has already occurred to your skin, evidenced by a leathery or mottled complexion with multiple brown spots or growths, begin its treatment by using a "richer" moisturizer and protecting against further damage. *Avoid the sun* and *use a SPF 15 sunblock* when exposure is unavoidable. We will discuss the correction of the other sequelae of sun injury in forthcoming chapters . . .

* * *

CHAPTER 3

Diet, Exercise and a Stable Weight

The most important factor in the diet is *water intake* since most of the water is delivered to the skin through the blood vessels. Except for patients with heart or kidney disease, at least one quart (4 glasses) of water is recommended daily to maintain the skin in a state of ideal hydration. This allows the skin to cleanse itself with healthy sweating and allows the skin cells to have normal turgor. Good, old-fashioned, inexpensive tap-water is generally best. Mineral waters are fine but should be of the *uncarbonated, low salt variety*. The salt content of some of the mineral waters encourages water-retention; the hardness and carbonation of others may favor kidney stones.

For most adults *at their ideal weights*, diets should be planned with approximately 1,800–2,000 calories if they have about average physical activity. This level of calories reflects the reduction in calorie allowances associated with advancing age proposed by the *National Research Council*. The general daily diet pattern should be planned with the Basic Four Food Groups (milk, meat, vegetable-fruit, and bread-cereal) as a guide.

For a well-balanced daily diet, portions from each of these good groups should be proportioned as follows:

(1) The *Milk Group* should include 1 glass for adults and 2 glasses for children and adolescents.

(2) The *Meat Group* (meat, fish, fowl, eggs, cheese) should consist of 2 servings.

(3) The *Vegetable-fruit Group* should comprise 4 daily servings. One Serving each day should consist of a dark green or a yellow vegetable for Vitamin A; one serving should consist of a citrus or other fruit rich in Vitamin C.

(4) The *Bread-cereal Group* should contribute 4 or more servings consisting of bread, cereal or potato.

Fats, desserts and additional servings of basic foods supplement the diet. Diets should be planned with *40% or less of the total calories from fat.* It is preferable to follow recommendations for a *low cholesterol, low saturated fatty acid diet* to keep the blood vessels to the skin unclogged as well as to the heart and brain. This requires substituting buttermilk or skim milk for whole milk, cottage cheese for other cheeses, and egg whites for whole eggs. Pork, ham, shellfish, and fish canned in oil should also be omitted although Canadian bacon and leg of lamb are allowed. The eating of fats such as butter and mayonnaise should be limited. Egg noodles, vegetables prepared with fat or cream, and avocado should be avoided. Intake of chocolate, nuts, olives and peanut butter should be minimized as well.

The well balanced diet contains all the vitamins and minerals most of us need. *Fresh vegetables and fruits* are best as vitamin sources. As a fail-safe against irregular eating habits, a *multi-vitamin* such as Theragran-M® is recommended and an *iron supplement* is suggested for menstruating women.

Exercise stimulates our circulation and keeps our "heart-lung machine" functioning well. A sluggish circulation results in fingers that turn cold quickly and a skin without the rosy freshness of a healthy blood supply. Regular exercise three times a week not only keeps us alive longer and makes us feel more vigorous, but improves our complexions. More blood—with its oxygen, water and nutriments—reaches our skin and the healthy perspiration cleanses our pores. Warm, moist heat such as steam baths, *if not overdone* can also benefit the skin by encouraging this self-cleansing. Any exercise program should be *started gradually* and be *continued regularly.* A few sessions of overly-vigorous "working out" or jogging do little but increase your chances for a heart attack! Competitive types, in particular, should heed this warning! Anyone with a health problem should consult their physician *before* embarking upon any exercise program.

Much has been said about facial exercises for retaining a youthful appearance. In general, I don't believe they are very helpful—and indeed *may be harmful.* However, there are several *good* ones and quite a few to *avoid.* If you look in the mirror at your profile while you touch the back of your tongue to the roof of your mouth, you will note one particular position which raises your *hyoid*—the bone at the root of your tongue. This is particularly good for keeping a clean neckline. A second exercise to be practiced, while looking in the mirror, is to open your eyes widely—so all redundant skin is taken into the upper lid crease—but to do so *without raising your brow.* This is helpful in preventing upper eyelid bags. Two isometric exercises, also to be practiced before the mirror, that are helpful include: (1) raising your eyebrow without creasing your forehead; and (2) raising the corners of your mouth without making a laughline crease. These "tone" up the muscles without encouraging wrinkles.

There are numerous exercises and habitual expressions that can be very harmful. Pursing your lips, as a smoker does when inhaling, contributes to the fine lines radiating from your lips *(perioral rhytides).* Clenching the teeth while grimacing and lowering the lower lip with the neck muscles *(platysma)*—as in an expression of disgust—can contribute to unattractive neck bands. Scowl lines, deep creases above eyebrows that are repetitively arched in speaking, and crow's feet worsened by habitual squinting may be minimized by noting customary facial over-animations that are above what we need for speech emphasis. While we don't want a "dead-pan" or expressionless visage, we don't need our eyebrows oscillating like those of Groucho Marx!

No two people will require the same amount of sleep. We all know how much—or how little—of it is required for us to look good and feel well. Suffice it to say that we should regularly strive for this amount. Most adults need between 6 and 8 hours of sleep nightly to feel well-rested. It is best if we sleep *on our backs with our heads elevated slightly* on a pillow. This allows gravity to work *for us* while we sleep—lessening puffy eyelids and not creasing in a jowl in the favorite side on which we sleep.

Think of the skin as a rubber band . . . If you expand and contract it many times, it eventually thins, frays and breaks. It looses its elasticity. The skin does this all by itself; we don't need to speed the process! Constantly putting on 10 to 15 pounds and then crash-dieting to take them off is very harmful to the skin. The rubber band gives out, and we are left with wrinkles and redundant folds of skin. We should try to retain a lean weight throughout our lives. That way, the few extra pounds we put on—as our amount of exercise and our metabolic rates decrease with age—will "take up the slack" to retain our youthful, wrinkle-free appearances. *The up and down weight gyrations of binge-eating followed by fad dieting are not only hazardous to your health in general, but abysmal for your skin!*

Weight should be removed gradually, no more than 15 pounds being removed in a month unless under direct Doctor's supervision. Just as rapid weight gain is accompanied by stretch marks or *striae*, rapid weight loss is accompanied by redundant skin that does not contract in all but the extremely young. It is also very important that essential minerals, vitamins and hydration be maintained during periods of weight-reduction. Like most problems, it is *better avoided than treated* and physician's supervision is suggested for any weight loss over 15 pounds.

The best way to lose weight and *keep it off* is to merely *reduce the size of your portions.* Fill your stomach with fluids—water—before eating and *eat slightly less—consistently.* Lower the 40% of fats to 20% or 30% and get accustomed to passing up the *fettucine, blini with Caviar* or *mousse au chocolate.* This develops a healthy style of eating that results in a stable weight which will not fluctuate wildly.

Alcohol, nicotine and excess caffeine all have deleterious effects upon the skin. Alcohol not only dehydrates you but causes a *vasodilation* (flushing) and *hypertrophy* (growth) of the sebaceous glands. It gives a flushed, dowdy appearance; its effect on the skin is well illustrated by the alcoholic's large, fleshy nose or *rhinophyma.* Caffeine is found in tea as well as coffee and in many sodas as well. Nicotine and caffeine are vasoconstrictive drugs which lessen the skin's blood supply and dehydrate you as well. Nicotine should be avoided and caffeine intake minimized. These are powerful drugs which have systemic effects far beyond the skin.

It is well to note that during periods of forced weight gain—such as an actor putting on weight for a part, during pregnancy, or while nursing—the skin should be *especially well-moisturized.* The enlarging stomach and breasts need the benefit of a rich moisturizer with Vitamin E to help prevent stretch marks *(striae)* from developing.

Any planned weight loss should ideally be *before* any "lifting" surgery so it will not create new wrinkles to be removed. While breasts show weight gain and loss, they do not show it to the same extent as the face and the rest of the body; the breast fat remains rather "sequestered" in a separate pool and is not *as* sensitive to weight fluctuations. After a "tuck" or "lifting" procedure, when the skin has been tightened and is under tension, a hypoallergenic, Vitamin E-enriched moisturizer is especially indicated to protect the skin which is particularly vulnerable at this time.

The preceding suggestions provide a guide for maintaining the youthful, wrinkle-free lustre of the skin and keeping the plastic surgeon away as long as possible. A mnemonic for avoiding facial wrinkles can be stated simply: *Never gain nor lose a pound, never smile nor frown excessively, sleep flat on your back, and avoid the sun like the plague.* If you have varied from these tenets before reading this book, it would be well to stop inflicting further injury to your skin by following them now. *It's not too late!* We will deal with correcting the damage you may have already done in the chapters that follow . . .

* * *

CHAPTER 4

The System and Its Variations

From the preceding chapters, it is evident that the basic skin care system consists of a simple, *three step regimen* carried out *twice a day, everyday*. The three steps are: *cleansing (step 1), toning (step 2), and moisturizing (step 3)*. The night and day moisturizers are different in reflection of their different purposes.

It is well to re-emphasize that the hands should be washed before touching the face and that either a soapless cleanser or glycerine and rosewater soap is best for this purpose. Also, the wash cloth should be changed daily—it should be soft and of good quality. This is all the *exfoliation* (shedding) the skin needs—anything rougher may do more damage than good. During periods of active eruptions (adolescent acne, for example), it should be laundered after every use. Towels, too, should be changed frequently and preferably daily. *Keep your hands away from your face and you can keep your face away from the plastic surgeon's hands longer!*

Unless you are going to run to the plastic surgeon, dermatologist or cosmetologist every few weeks, it would be well to get to know your skin and recognize the times at which the regimen should be varied. The human organism is adapted to maintain *homeostasis*—a stable, relatively unchanging, internal environment. However, the outside world—the conditions to which we are exposed—varies constantly. The skin adapts well to most of these changes, but has limits to its adaptability. We should learn to vary our care to reflect the changing needs of the skin and to maintain that *homeostasis*.

For example, the simplest variation is the substitution of the clarifier for the toner in step 2 for one or both of the three step rituals. When beginning the system or for those with very oily skins, a clarifier is substituted for the toner in step 2. Those with oilier skin (Blacks in general) and younger men, in particular, may prefer to use the clarifier regularly, at least in the morning, or even in both performances of the regimen. It may be used in spot fashion for trouble areas. During periods when the skin is oilier—periods of stress and perhaps pre-menstrually—it may be well to cut back on the "richness" or frequency of moisturizer application. The Day moisturizer should still be used, but the night moisturizer may be temporarily omitted or a less rich one employed.

If you leave your make-up on overnight, something that should be avoided, I would recommend using the clarifier for step 2 the following day to keep the pores unblocked. The same is true if you switch to a heavier than usual make-up or wear it longer hours or more frequently—for example, during the Christmas party season.

There are multiple occasions in which a "richer" moisturizer should be employed; the night moisturizer should be the one changed. When spending a lot of time at the beach or on the tennis courts in the sun, the skin needs more moisturizing supplement than usual. When being chafed with windburns and sun on the skislopes, the skin not only needs a moisturizing sunscreen, but needs extra moisturization at night as well. The same requirement may also exist in the middle of Winter if the heating is dry hot air. *A bedroom humidifier is recommended as well to lessen this problem.* Its water should be changed regularly.

Do not forget that *sun exposure at the beach constitutes just a small fraction of the total exposure the skin receives* in our lives. It is constantly exposed to small amounts of actinic radiation everytime we are outdoors. The harmful effects are cumulative. The skin needs protection at these times as well with a sunscreen in the day moisturizer!

The extra necessity of protective moisturization during periods of weight gain (such as pregnancy or nursing) was emphasized in previous chapters. Switching to a richer night moisturizer and even temporary upgrading to a richer day moisturizer is indicated during these periods to protect the skin of the abdomen, breasts and face. Vitamin E in the moisturizer may help protect against *striae*.

After surgery, the skin is especially sensitive and vulnerable. The skin has been temporarily *denervated* (rendered with less-than-normal sensation and sweating ability) and cannot cleanse itself as well as normally. Cleasing must be especially thorough and gentle. A clarifier is indicated as are hypo-allergenic products and moisturizers with Vitamin E.

During periods of weight reduction—which as previously mentioned should be *gradual*—the skin can use extra moisturization. Moisturizers used should be richer to give the skin all the help it can get in shrinking to the leaner frame. Unfortunately, it only succeeds in the very young in adapting to marked or sudden weight losses.

Attempt to maintain homeostasis! Get your skin as blemish-free as possible with the basic system, and vary the system as needed to make up for changes in your environment. Keep your skin's environment the same—optimal. *Develop a definite SKIN-SENSE—get to know the needs of your skin!* If, after all is said and done, scars, growths, blemishes, or wrinkles remain, read on as we get to their treatment . . .

* * *

PART I
FACESAVING

B. Skin Smoothing—
Improving Damaged Skin

CHAPTER 5

Facemasks and Facials

F*acials* are a ticklish subject. Think of the skin as suspended by springy attachments to the bony prominences, particularly the cheek bones, the rims of the orbits, and the chin. Its attachments are loosened by time as the collagen and elastin fibrils in the skin degenerate. The harmful ultraviolet component of sunlight accelerates this change. These attachments are attenuated and loosened by stretching or pulling the skin in *any* direction—upwards and sideways, as well as down. You can't just manipulate the skin of the face up and have it *stay* up without surgery. Indeed, *aggressive manipulation of the facial skin is harmful!*

This consideration leads us to certain fears and warnings about facials. A gentle, cleansing facial which includes careful expression of the contents of some stubborn oil glands can be very stimulating to the skin and even beneficial. However, *adequate daily cleansing, occasional application of a clarifier, and use of a face mask should obviate the need for this treatment.* Repeated squeezings or application of suction must *inevitably* result in some permanent scarring, dilation of blood vessels *(telangiectasia)*, or blemish as the skin becomes more fragile with age. One not-so-gentle facial can do a great deal of damage.

For these reasons, *I cannot endorse facials but only warn about their possible hazards.* None-the-less, I cannot condemn a carefully performed and gentle facial, but only remind the reader that *consistent, adequate care of the skin should render it unnecessary.*

A *facemask* is a preparation designed to tighten the skin and cleanse it. There are two basic varieties: the peel-off type and the wash-off type. Of the two, I prefer the wash-off type because it is more gentle to the skin.

Facemasks are ideal for minimizing fine wrinkles and absorbing impurities from the skin. They are particularly good for oily skin. Normal skin can benefit from application of a mask once weekly or before a special evening or event. Since a good mask is very absorbent, oily skins should employ the mask more frequently.

Masks should be applied after first cleansing the face. They are generally to be left on 10 to 15 minutes to have their "tightening" effects. I prefer the *kaolin* variety for its particular absorbancy. They are particularly effective if applied *warm (not hot)*, for they open the pores for deeper cleansing. They should be rinsed off with cool water; a toner should be applied afterwards.

Although the effect they have on wrinkles may be just a temporary one, it can be very flattering for that special evening. They are most useful in primarily *deep-cleaning* the skin to help avoid blackheads and whiteheads. They do this *gently* without requiring any rough manipulation of the skin.

I recommend *once-weekly* application of a wash-off kaolin mask to most patients and more frequent—twice or even three times a week—application for people with oilier skin types or difficult-to-clear-up eruptions. I believe a good mask can be a straight arrow in the quiver of skin treatment, keeping the plastic surgeon away for just a little longer.

* * *

CHAPTER 6

Removing Blemishes

The vast majority of the innumerable growths and discolorations we commonly refer to as blemishes may be removed in the office or ignored. However, a few require more aggressive treatment. Unfortunately, it usually takes an educated eye to differentiate between them. In what follows, I present guidelines to the recognition and treatment of common problems, organized into categories based upon treatment. Acne scars merit an entire chapter on their treatment and are dealt with separately in the next chapter.

A. BLEMISHES BEST LEFT ALONE

Freckles *(ephilides)* are benign, flat or punctate collections of tan to brown pigment. More common in redheads and more prominent in adolescence, they are *intensified by sun exposure and gradually regress with age.* Protecting the skin with sunscreens during the day and a sunblock when in direct sunlight can substantially reduce their noticeability.

The age spot, or *lentigo senilis*, is a flat patch of brown pigmentation occurring anywhere on the body, but most often on the back of the hands and the face in older individuals. These are benign, but are *intensified by continued sun exposure.* Besides protecting your skin with a sunscreen during the day and a sunblock at the beach, I recommend you apply a *Fade Cream* with *hydroquinone* at night to the affected areas. Although there is a low incidence of hypersensitivity reactions to this bleaching agent, many of these age spots respond well over a period of 3 to 6 weeks. If an irritation develops, or if there is no response to the fade cream, a *light dermabrasion* may be successful in removing them.

B. BLEMISHES BEST REMOVED WITHOUT SURGERY

Spiders or *telangiectasias* are small, stellate blemishes with a reddish hue from the capillary blood within them, representing dilations or small connections between blood vessels. They temporarily disappear with pressure and result from noticed or inadvertent trauma in older individuals. *Rough handling of the skin can cause these blemishes!* The best treatment is *needle-point electrodesiccation of the feeding blood vessels at the center.* This is a painless office procedure that may be easily repeated if the first attempt at removal is unsuccessful.

Warts *(Verrucae vulgaris)* are common roughened and raised growths occurring in children as well as adults. Usually caused by a virus, they are contagious and can be spread from one part of the body to another. They appear most often on the hands and feet. Regressing twice as often in boys than in girls, two-thirds disappear in two years. *Electrodesiccation is the best treatment*; the projection of the wart may be burned away under local anesthesia and the fragments scraped away. Surgery and application of caustics are less frequently successful.

C. BLEMISHES REQUIRING SURGICAL REMOVAL

Pigmented moles or *nevi* are mostly benign, their removal being solely cosmetic. The "beauty spot" on the cheek is a common example. The more infantile type *(junctional nevi)* are usually flat, hairless and smooth; the adult type *(intradermal nevi)* are usually raised, hairy and rough. If the infantile type persists into adulthood, a *melanoma* may result. This malignancy will be discussed later. A large percentage of moles occurring on the face have a junctional component. Therefore *with any occurrence of bleeding, itching, change in size or pigmentation, removal is recommended.* Most of these are *amenable to office excision under local anesthesia.* Non-surgical methods, such as desiccation and application of caustics are to be *condemned* for frequent failure to eradicate all the neval cells and for possibly inciting malignant change in residual cells.

In the adult, *sun abuse and aging are causes of two categories of keratoses*, emphasizing the importance of protecting the skin from the sun. The first, *senile keratoses*, do have malignant potential; their removal is usually justified to differentiate them from skin carcinomas. They appear as raised, scaly lesions on exposed areas such as the face and hands after many years of sun-worshipping. Most of these are *amenable to office excision* under local anesthesia. Large areas of involvement may be treated with topical applications of 5-*Fluorouracil cream* under the direction of a physician. The second category, *sebhorrheic keratoses*, consists of waxy, "tacked on" growths of no malignant potential. They usually are *excised in the office for purely cosmetic reasons* or for assurance that they are not more serious growths.

Two skin malignancies *caused by sun damage* are the *basal cell* and *squamous carcinoma*. The former is a waxy, discreet nodule of grey, yellow or pink color which tends to bleed on slight injury. As it grows, basal cell cancer tends to ulcerate in the center and develop a characteristic rolled edge. The tumor is scaly or crusty and may be pigmented. Untreated, it slowly and continuously erodes through underlying structures earning it the nickname of *rodent ulcer*. A more rapidly-growing skin malignancy is *squamous cell carcinoma*. It has a propensity for affecting the lower lip and is *associated with pipe and cigarette smoking*. Although it may grossly appear very similar to the basal cell, there is a greater degree of surrounding firmness. Squamous cell carcinomas may originate in forms similar to the keratoses from which they are derived. They may spread to nearby lymph nodes. *Treatment of both is surgical excision* with complete removal demonstrated by pathological examination of the margins of the excision. Most small skin cancers can be treated in the office. For larger ones, skin grafting or techniques of shifting adjacent or remote tissue may be required. Complete removal allowing pathologic examination and judgment of the adequacy of surgery is essential. The lymph nodes are not treated unless there is evidence of involvement.

Melanoma is the dreaded black cancer occurring in a nevus or in the pigmented coat of the eye. It may occur anywhere in the body and can spread quickly to lymph nodes and elsewhere. *Any nevus which is noticed to change in size, height, or color, which ulcerates, bleeds or becomes tender should be suspect.* Peripheral smaller pigmented spots surrounding a larger one are *very* suspicious. The first change is likely to be increased pigmentation. Typically a melanoma is blue-black or brown, firm, smooth and non-hairy. It may be small in size, from an eighth of an inch to several inches in diameter with irregular borders. Diagnosis is by *excisional biopsy*, that is, cutting out the entire growth. If this biopsy is positive, a *wide surgical excision* under general anesthesia is indicated with removal of the nearby lymph nodes for deeper forms of the disease.

Hutchinson's melanotic freckle *(lentigo maligna)* is a pigmented freckle with irregular borders and variegated pigmentation. Usually larger than half an inch and characteristically occurring on the face, it frequently *precedes clinical melanoma*. It *should be excised*, although excision need not be radical.

Sebaceous and *epidermal inclusion cysts*, *lipomas*, and *fibromas* are benign swellings presenting as unsightly or slightly tender lumps just beneath the skin. Treatment is *elective surgical excision.* A small ellipse of overlying skin must be included when removing cysts. Usually this may be done under local anesthesia as an office procedure.

* * * *

NOTE: Interested readers may find a more complete listing and detailed discussion of "Birthmarks, Skin and Subcutaneous Tumors" in Chapter VI of *The Kindest Cut* by the same author.

* * *

CHAPTER 7

Eradicating Acne Scars

We humans are inferior to several lower forms of life in our healing capacities. Whereas salamanders can regenerate a limb identical to the original, we can only repair injury by creation of *scar tissue*. Scar is an inferior substitute for the original skin which it replaces. It is not as strong, has a different texture and color, and has several other undesireable features.

Scars, whether caused by acne, chickenpox or trauma, have several properties which draw visual attention. They may be *broad* because healing occurred in a delayed fashion *(secondary intention)* or in the presence of infection. They are usually of a *different color*. Initially, most scars are red and raised, earning them the nickname of "proud flesh". As a normal scar matures, it blanches, flattens and fades in color. The *color of the scar usually contrasts sharply and abruptly* with surrounding, normal skin. The scar is usually *different in height* from the surrounding skin. Fresh scars are usually raised, later on they are usually depressed. This is particularly true of acne scars; the rims of these crater-like depressions usually have *sharp borders* which cast shadows that accentuate the skin's imperfections. Scars may also *cross lines of facial expression* or *interfere with the free mobility of the skin* during facial animation. Since we cannot make scars into normal skin, we must remove as many of the reasons for which we notice them as possible!

We can cut out or *excise* a broad scar or particularly deep acne sinus. The short, slender surgical scar may be much less noticeable that the broader scar or deep pit which preceded it. By techniques which shift its direction, such as *Z-plasty* or *W-plasty*, we can *revise* a scar so it does not interfere with facial expression and is thus less noticeable.

By local injections of steroids *(Kenalog®)*, we can make a scar mature faster so that it will lighten in color sooner. This is particularly good for markedly-raised and angry-looking scars which may be termed *hypertrophic* and scars that overgrow the margins of the original injury and are termed *keloids*. Blacks are particularly prone to this latter problem.

We can make the change in color from the scar to normal skin less abrupt by *dermabrasion*. The top layer of the skin is sanded away with a rotating wheel, brush or fraise. By dermabrading with a fine diamond burr, the sides of the crater may be made less vertical, so that the shadows cast are not as severe. There is a less abrupt change in height in the skin—making the scar less noticeable. Dermabrasion is best in the fairer skin types because the skin color is usually lightened to some degree. For this reason, the face is usually dermabraded in "aesthetic units" consisting of the upper lip and muzzle area between laughlines, from the laughlines to upper borders of the cheekbones, and the forehead. After having a dermabrasion, most patients will *sunburn easier and will not tan as well.* As if the innumerable ones mentioned earlier were not enough, they will have an additional reason to protect their skin!

Dermabrasion is readily performed as an office procedure under local anesthesia. This has been facilitated by the use of a *Hydron®* dressing, originally designed for use in burn units, which eases the care of dermabraded patients. I apply it as a paste to the freshly dermabraded skin, keeping the wound sealed and sterile. Unlike cumbersome gauze dressings, it rapidly polymerizes as a see-through face mask. The patient is virtually *pain-free* as healing takes place rapidly beneath it with much less of the discomfort and "weeping" that accompanied other types of dressings. When healing is complete in 5 to 8 days, it peels off easily in a warm shower.

We can "plump" up a depressed scar or deep acne pit with injectable collagen *(Zyderm®)* so that the scar is level with the surrounding skin. Collagen is to the body as steel girders are to a skyscraper. It comprises 83% of the skin and bone. With the exception of those with rare auto-immune diseases, no one is allergic to collagen itself. However, there is a very low incidence of sensitivity to the solution in which it must be dissolved for injection. Therefore *a skin test is done first.* If this is negative, treatments are usually scheduled at 3 to 4 week intervals, until the final result is achieved. The total amount required can be estimated after the first treatment and varies significantly from patient to patient.

For mild cases of acne scarring, either dermabrasion or *Zyderm®* injections provide good correction. The more olive the complexion, the greater is my preference for *Zyderm®*. For only a few scattered acne pits, I favor excision and *Zyderm®*. Excision of deep pits is performed under local anesthesia in the office and is facilitated by the use of a *fine dermal punch* which resembles a very fine cork-borer. One or two sutures suffice to close each site.

For more severe cases of acne scaring, I prefer to begin with a dermabrasion and then "touch up" any remaining imperfections with *Zyderm®*. This allows a more rapid correction and requires fewer treatments. A second dermabrasion may offer additional improvement.

Severe acne scarring may be accompanied by such a loss of skin tone that a dowdy look with premature jowling may result—even in very young individuals. In these patients, cheeklift *(meloplasty)* may be indicated *before* any of the above-mentioned procedures can be implemented. This procedure will be discussed in later chapters.

Since dermabrasion may temporarily block the pores with dead cellular debris, it is important to use *gentle clarifiers* in the skin care regimen as soon as the *Hydron®* dressing is removed. Since make-up will probably be required to camouflage the temporary redness which persists from 3 to 6 weeks, it should be hypoallergenic and *removed carefully and completely at night with a gentle, soapless cleanser.* A *moisturizer is essential* to help this redness fade rapidly. It is also preferable to upgrade the direct-sun protection to a *SPF 12-15 sunblock.*

Like silk, skin is a precious and fragile fabric; once damaged, its original state is difficult, if not impossible, to restore. Therefore, *proper skin care is important to prevent these problems.* However, when they are present, by a combination of techniques described above, *80 to 90% correction can be achieved with acne scars.* While this is substantial, it is still less than 100%. Fortunately, we sometimes do a little better, and good make-up can compensate for the residual 5–10%.

CHAPTER 8

Rejuvenating the Skin

As skin ages, it loses its protective moisturizers, dries out and becomes leathery. It becomes thinner and more fragile. Fine wrinkles begin to lace its surface, crossing the lines of facial expression as streets cross a major avenue. Wrinkles are born that radiate from the corners of the eyes as crow's feet and the vermilion borders of the lips.

These fine wrinkles or *rhytides* are more pronounced and occur earlier in those who have not followed the suggestions made in previous chapters in their younger years. However, do not despair . . . Something can be done to improve the situation.

When there are only a few fine wrinkles it is possible to eliminate them by filling up the creases with injectable collagen. This is the same *Zyderm*® preparation discussed in the previous chapter for acne scars. Per routine, *a skin test is performed first* and treatments scheduled 3–4 weeks apart. For a few fine, early wrinkles, one or two treatments usually suffice.

When there are too many wrinkles to be treated by injection, we must employ another means to remedy the situation. A *chemical peel* may be performed, usually in the office. A *phenol* solution is generally chosen to give the facial skin a superficial burn. The solution is applied under local anesthesia with premedication to counteract the light burning sensation that occurs. Only "aesthetic units" are peeled. This consists of either the entire face or the upper lip and "muzzle" area of the face between the laughlines, the cheeks between laughlines and the upper borders of the cheekbones, or the forehead. The solution is "feathered" beneath the lower border of the jaw. The neck is *not* peeled because it is prone to scarring.

It is desireable that the patient speak and chew as little as possible during the first 72 hours after the peel when the patient should just relax at home. Two weeks need be set aside from work or social activity.

After the facial skin recovers from this first degree burn in 5–8 days, a wonderful thing will have happened. The collagen fibrils, the networking support system of the skin, will lose their "memory". Rather than being organized *parallel* to the old wrinkles, they will come back in a *random*, criss-cross pattern with *obliteration of these finer wrinkles*.

However, there is a small trade-off to be made for the elimination of these fine wrinkles. Some of the pigment cells or *melanocytes* are damaged by the peel so that *the complexion usually becomes a little lighter*. The patient will be likely to *sun burn easier* and *may not tan as well*. It is advisable to *avoid the sun for 6 weeks unless a total sunblock is used*. Afterwards, the skin will require extra protection in the sun with a *SPF 12-15 sunblock*.

During the healing period, a temporary redness may persist from 3 to 6 weeks. This can be easily camouflaged with make-up which should be *carefully and completely removed at night with a soapless cleanser*. As with dermabrasion, a *gentle clarifier* is indicated for several weeks afterwards to keep the pores unblocked from cellular debris, and *moisturizing* is essential to help the redness fade rapidly.

When there are innumerable deep wrinkles radiating from the vermilion borders of the lips—as in habitual lip pursers or heavy smokers (from drawing on the cigarette), dermabrasion of the "muzzle" area may be superior to a peel. The rotating burr or drum, under a surgeon's direct vision and control, can better even out the inequalities of skin height about these wrinkles. Also, any brown spots that have not responded to the *fade cream with hydroquinone* may be dermabraded at the same time. The rest of the face may be peeled in routine fashion. I will generally apply the *Hydron*® dressing described in the last chapter to any dermabraded areas to ensure patient comfort.

Dermabrasions and chemical peels change the skin *permanently*. However, the clock will tick on and new wrinkles may form. Similarly new wrinkles may form next to those that were eliminated with *Zyderm*® or old ones may eventually reform under continued identical stresses. Dermabrasion and chemical peels may be repeated to achieve further improvement after several years. *Zyderm*® injections can be continued indefinitely.

Those with darker skins and deep olive complexions are not good candidates for either dermabrasion or chemical peels because of the pigment abnormalities that may result. I will usually "tide them over" with *Zyderm®* injections before resorting to lifting surgery. Fortunately, pulling the skin taut tends to flatten out fine wrinkles as well as the coarse ones for which it is primarily indicated. *The neck cannot be safely dermabraded or peeled;* it can only be treated with *Zyderm®* until it is time for a necklift, which brings us to the next section . . .

* * *

PART I
FACESAVING

C. Skinshaping—
Taking Up the Excess

CHAPTER 9

Eyelid Lifts

The eyes vie with the mouth for supremacy as the most expressive feature on the face. In conversation, we focus on each other's eyes. Being called the "mirror to the soul", the eyes are generally indicative of a person's alertness, happiness or unhappiness and frequently suggest the previous evening's pursuits. Problems arise when the eyes are sending messages contradictory to actual feelings. This frequently becomes a concern when we develop sagging eyelids, dark rings or pouches under our eyes which suggest an evening of debauchery when we were alone in our bed at 10:00.

As we age, a redundancy of upper lid skin develops and becomes crepey as the skin's attachments to the underlying muscle loosen. An unsightly fold creeps down over the upper lid and may even overlap the lashes. This fold continues toward the temple into multiple, deep crow's feet that persist even when we are not smiling. The skin of the lower lid becomes redundant as well and gives us a sagging, tired look, which is present even after a good night's sleep. Our eyes appear to get smaller, the lids may droop, and the field of vision is decreased in marked cases. Although this is usually the result of age, the condition is sometimes inherited, making even a teenager or young adult look overly weary and older than necessary. When this occurs, it is usually accompanied by either marked eyelid allergies, extra fat, or a prominence of the upper, outer portion of the eye socket.

Removing these traces of age has a remarkable rejuvenating effect on appearance. The technique is called *blepharoplasty* or an "eyelid lift". My patients have often told me that friends who did not know about their surgery commented on "how relaxed", "how well-rested", or "how good" they looked

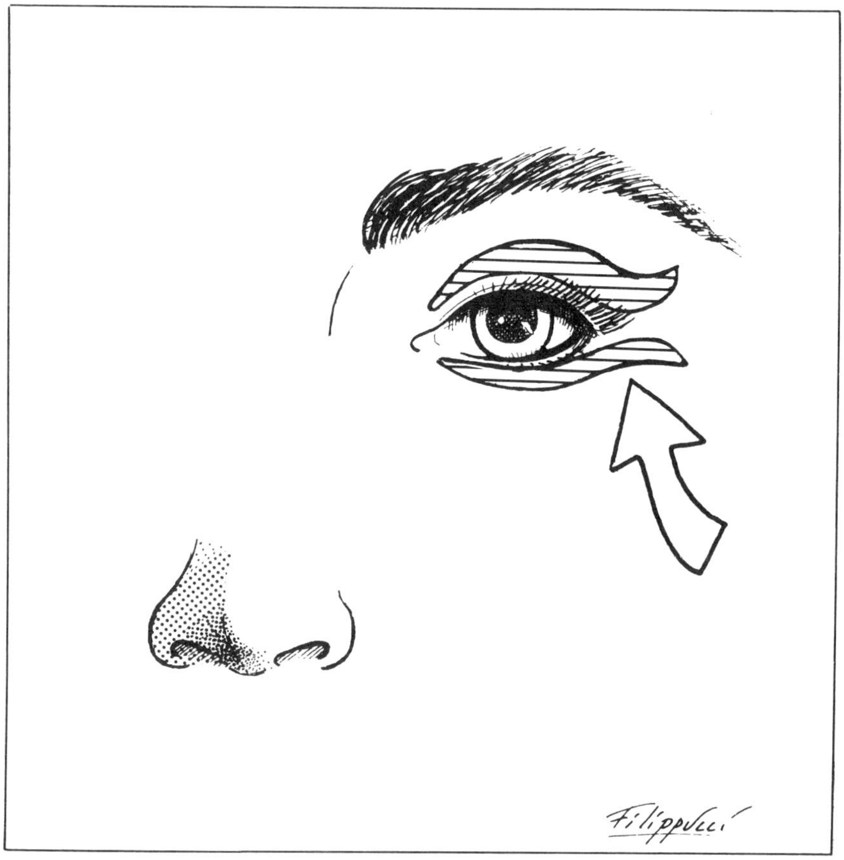

FIGURE 1: A typical "fish-tailed", elliptical pattern of redundant upper and lower eyelid skin is shown for removal in eyelid lift (*blepharoplasty*).

afterwards without being able to specifically pinpoint why they looked different. This is common because none of the fundamental features of the face are altered. Depending on your age and skin condition, the younger look achieved can be expected to last for 5 to 10 years.

In performing a *blepharoplasty*, redundant skin from the lids is removed in modified elliptical patterns and wedges as illustrated (See **Fig. 1**). The skin heals very rapidly and all sutures may be removed by the third or fourth day. The patient need only wear tinted glasses for 7–10 days and a very rapid return to social life is possible; any residual bruising resolves during the next week and can be covered with make-up.

CASE HISTORIES

While the experiences most patients have with eyelid lifts might best be exemplified simply by the print model M. B. who needed less "air brushing" after surgery and got sent on younger "go sees", two other patients who had particularly gratifying experiences are described below.

C. M. was a 48-year-old housewife unhappy with increasing bagginess and crepiness around her eyes, who became depressed at the prospect of her daughter's marriage. She saw that event as meaning that she was "over the hill". Determined to fight those feelings, she consulted me and had an eyelid lift under local anesthesia in the office, followed by collagen injections to eliminate vertical frown lines between her eyebrows. She was delighted with her more alert and happier look, which enhanced her own naturally high cheek bones and well-kept skin. "I don't look like a tired, angry old lady anymore." She proudly and confidently breezed through her daughter's wedding looking younger than her son-in-law's mother. Afterwards she went on to enter the business world for the first time in her life since "the nest was now empty."

R.W., in contrast, was a 45-year-old salesman in a rut on a job he had held for over 20 years. He just never seemed to be able to get anywhere. He knew his unhappiness was taking a toll on his job performance. Yet whenever he looked in the mirror, he saw an aging man who should be slowing down. After eyelid lift, his energy and enthusiasm returned and he took off like a house on fire. Within 7 months, he was offered a promotion to regional manager with substantial raise. Shortly thereafter, he was able to buy a house and move his family to a desireable suburb.

PREPARATION

Blepharoplasty is one of the most ideal procedures for local anesthesia and outpatient, office surgery. I usually prescribe *Vitamin C* and *Vitamin K* preoperatively to optimize healing and minimize bruising respectively. *Vitamin E* and *aspirin-containing drugs* should be avoided for 2 weeks prior to surgery. Aspirin interferes with the blood's ability to clot. *Tylenol*® is an over-the-counter analgesic that may be used instead. On the day of surgery, the face is washed with *Phisohex*® to eliminate troublesome bacteria and *no make-up, false eyelashes or contact lens are worn.*

When you arrive at the office, you will undress and put on a hospital gown. Then you are premedicated with injections. After they have taken effect, you will be brought into the Operating Room. A needle is inserted into a vein in your arm and attached to a bottle of sugar water which drips slowly into you; this is called an *intravenous* and facilitates administration of sedatives and relaxants during surgery. The surgery itself takes about an hour and a half, followed by resting in the Recovery Room with iced saline compresses for a few hours and a gentle return home wearing sunglasses to conceal sutures.

If you prefer hospitalization—mandatory if you choose *general anesthesia*—you arrive the day before surgery and usually stay only two nights. Eyelid surgery, when performed *alone* in healthy patients, is more frequently performed in the office than in the hospital. It is also much more frequently performed under local anesthesia than general because it is advantageous to have the patient able to cooperate when the surgeon does the lower lids.

THE PROCEDURE

I believe the real work of the surgeon in eyelid lifting occurs *not when he picks up the scalpel, but ten minutes earlier.* That's when I use a skin marker which looks something like a felt tip pen. I carefully draw on the upper lid the area of skin to be removed. I check the effect this will have using a blunt-edged tweezer to pinch the skin along the lines of the planned incision. This "testing" assures me that I will remove enough skin to get the desired effect, but not too much—which would prevent the eye from closing properly. It also guarantees that the incision will be properly placed to disappear inconspicuously into the eyelid crease. Then, noting the natural skin crease caused by smiling, I draw the outer portion of lower lid incision. The amount of skin to be removed here is not determined until later during surgery.

After the face is painted with a surgical cleanser, I inject high-concentration local anesthesia into the eyelid with a very fine gauge needle. I tell my patients that it will feel like a mosquito bite, because I want them to be prepared for a different sensation. But not one has ever called it much to say "ouch" about. Remember, this this time you are floating away on pre-medications and intravenous relaxants.

In performing a *blepharoplasty* for skin redundancy *(blepharochalasis)*, I cut along the upper lid lines I have drawn and then carefully remove the excess skin from the underlying muscle. There is very little bleeding, but what little occurs is immediately stopped by the use of *electrocautery*. A fine wand is used which delivers small bursts of current to seal off tiny arteries. Not only does this provide a clear surgical field, but it minimizes later bruising.

Then I place four or five individual stitches of very fine thread to align the skin, and finish with a running stitch all along the incision line. This line falls in the natural fold of the eyelid and ends in the natural "smile" creases above the outer corner of the eye. After repeating this process on the other upper lid, I am ready to move to the lower lids.

After cutting along the outer portion of the lower lid incision with a scalpel, I use very delicate scissors beneath the lashes to assure that none are cut. The skin is separated from the underlying muscle. Then I ask my patient to open his or her mouth as wide as possible. This permits me to see how much skin is drawn down over the cheek when the person is speaking or yawning. If the surgeon skips this step, the lower lid may turn away from the eyeball giving an unattractive, sad look. In this case, the eye would be round instead of almond-shaped and too much white would show beneath the iris *(inferior scleral show)*. Any excess skin is lifted upward and outward and then is cut away. The outer portion is sewn with interrupted stitches and the incision under the lashes is closed with a running stitch.

The process is repeated on the other lower lid. Finally, I apply an anti-bacterial ophthalmic ointment to the suture lines; and iced water compresses are immediately placed on the eyelids.

RECUPERATION

After office surgery, you continue the cold compresses at home for several days, and apply the ophthalmic ointment to the suture lines at least three times a day. Prescriptions also are provided for a mild analgesic to alleviate

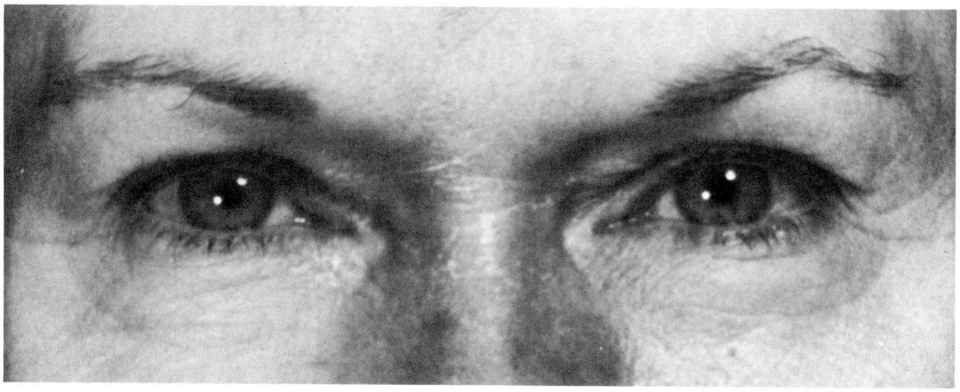

PHOTO 1: A patient with redundant skin of her upper and lower eyelids and lower eyelid bags.

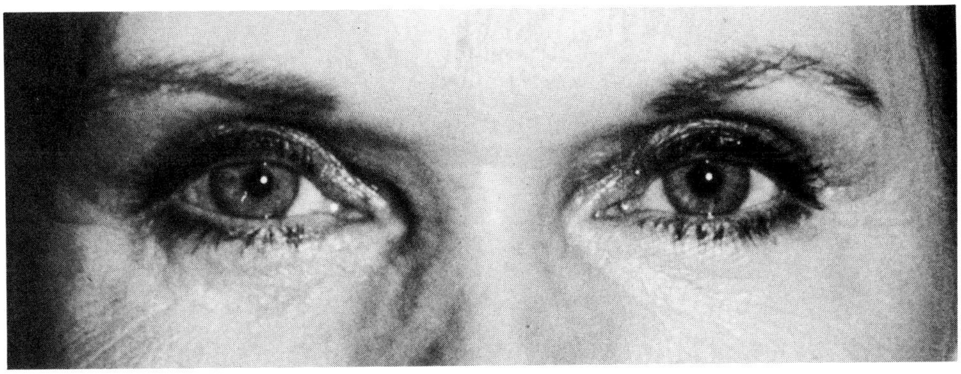

PHOTO 2: The same patient after eyelid lift *(blepharoplasty)* in which redundant skin and fat was removed.

any minimal discomfort and for lubricating eye drops to abate any "scratchy" or dry feeling which might occur. It usually is not comfortable to read for the first two or three days after surgery but pain is very rare.

Skin around the eye heals very rapidly. By the third or fourth day after surgery, you return to the office for suture removal which feels like a little tugging and pulling in a sensitive area but is not painful. You probably will want to continue wearing tinted glasses socially, because *it is not advisable to begin wearing make-up until four days after suture removal.* Then I recommend only hypoallergenic make-up and recommend its *complete and gentle removal at night with a soapless cleanser* applying it *only with the hands* and *in the direction of the incisions*, from inside to out. A *moisturizer with Vitamin E* is recommended to facilitate healing.

Within 10 days to two weeks from surgery, any residual bruising should be resolved and your eyes should look "normal" again, although more rested. Occasionally, some patients find that minor residual swelling persists for an additional week or two. A typical result of *blepharoplasty* is shown in **Photos 1** and **2**.

After blepharoplasty, you should *avoid heavy sun exposure for at least 6 weeks* because of the sun's effect of increasing swelling in operated areas. A sunburn is a first degree burn; it is an insult to the skin, as is surgery itself. The effects exacerbate each other. Should direct and prolonged sun exposure by unavoidable within the first 6 weeks, dark sunglasses and a total sunblock are mandatory.

PRECAUTIONS AND POTENTIAL PROBLEMS

If you have dry or scratchy eyes, I will refer you to an ophthalmologist before *blepharoplasty*. You should be aware that any tendency toward dry eyes may be made temporarily worse by surgery. However, this brief period can be eased by the use of synthetic tears available over the counter at pharmacies.

Certain "standard" surgical risks are *concomitant to all surgery* and eyelid surgery is no exception. These include *bleeding, infection* and *scarring.* Any bleeding that occurs during surgery is controlled at that time; if it occurs later, any collection of blood *(hematoma)* is easily evacuated. The result to the patient is usually only bruising that persists a few days longer. Infection occurs very seldom in facial surgery but would be controlled with appropriate antibiotics. The eyelids are fortunate in that bad scarring is seldom found in this area, even in Blacks who are prone to bad scarring in other areas. However, any objectionable scar may be subsequently revised or dermabraded easily as a minor procedure if this is necessary.

Two problems may occasionally be seen *specifically in blepharoplasty*. Occasionally, small inclusion cysts called *milia* form around the suture lines several weeks after surgery. They can be expressed by the surgeon in his office, much like whiteheads, with little discomfort. They can be avoided by *gentle cleaning twice daily with a gentle cleanser*. Even less frequently, tearing develops from a slight turning away of the eye or loss of contact with the lower lid. This is usually caused by postoperative swelling. It is almost always temporary and can be eased with a supporting adhesive steristrip worn for a week or two. If the problem does not resolve, it is called an *ectropion*, and a small office adjustment can be made to remedy the situation permanently.

JUST BLEPHAROPLASTY?

If you are considering any other facial plastic surgery, an eye lift may provide the added touch you are seeking. In practice, I frequently do eyelid lifting in conjunction with a cheek, full face or forehead lift, cheek augmentation, or with nasal reprofiling. Concurrent face or cheek lift allows the removal of a greater amount of lower eyelid skin for an even more positive final result. It facilities elimination of the cheek hollows *(nasojugal folds)* that occur beneath lower eyelid bags as does cheek augmentation with an implant inserted through the lower lid incision. A broad nasal bridge detracts markedly from the eyes; they look more "alert" without a wide "divider" separating them. Eyebrow sagging is always at least partly responsible for the redundancy of upper lid skin; a forehead lift corrects this aspect of the problem directly.

I am often asked whether plastic surgery can actually change the shape of the eye, and the answer is *yes*. "Round" eyes can be changed to "almond" eyes; small, downcast eyes can be changed to more open, "happier" eyes; droppy eyelids can be lifted; oriental eyes can be "Westernized"; eyelid bags and festoons can be eliminated. These procedures require surgery upon the deeper tissues—the fat, muscles, cartilage, or bone—which is performed through the above-described skin incisions before closure. They are dealt with in the sections which follow . . .

CHAPTER 10

Face and Necklifts

The goal of growing old gracefully might have been conceived and thought possible when people died in plagues or battles before the age of 30 or 40, but now that we actually live 70 or 80 years, the ravages of time may make this goal very elusive. The long term effects of gravity upon the face, the loss of skin elasticity with age, and the innumerable smiles and frowns, accentuated by the effects of sun-worship and marked weight fluctuation, result in the marked wrinkles associated with age. In the Orient, such wrinkles are accompanied by respectful treatment and reverence; but in Western countries, particularly the U.S., where a youthful ideal is maintained, such changes in appearance meet with reactions like "He's too old to run for President!" or "She danced spectacularly—and at her age!"

Just as the skin of the eyelids becomes crepey as its attachments to the underlying muscle loosen, similar changes occur in the face. The facial skin is more firmly attached to the rims of the orbits, the cheek bones, the mastoid area behind the ears, and the mid-portion of the face. As these attachments loosen, the cheek skin sags downward as if it were the middle of a hammock weighted by a person's derriere. An unattractive hollow *(nasojugal fold)* is created beneath a lower eyelid bag which gives the face a fatigued appearance. Laughlines *(nasolabial folds)* deepen and a height difference appears between the mouth and cheek area as the bone about the teeth recedes. As sagging skin overlaps the jawline, a jowl develops and may even extend into a dewlap.

As the neck skin becomes crepey and saggy, the sharp and crisp angle between the neck and the jaw is obscured. Unattractive vertical bands may develop and web the neck. Much like rings around a tree trunk, circumferential wrinkles multiply and encircle the neck. Double or triple chins may develop.

In the early part of the century, "minitucks" originated in France and Germany. These were essentially small scalp excisions resulting in temporary improvement. They led to the development of lifting procedures utilizing S-shaped incisions in the hairline and undermining akin to current techniques for "skin only" facelifts to achieve more permanent results. More recently, attention has been directed to the forehead, underlying fat, fascia, muscles, and bony prominences to further prolong and enhance results.

These operations are particularly sought by those who desire to work and socialize in their later years and wish to look as vital and energetic as they feel, without being prematurely stereotyped into the rocking-chair generation. In the business world, they are also sought by those in middle years who want to maintain the "competitive edge" over their younger rivals. *They are more and more frequently sought by everyday people—like you and me—who just wish to look as good as possible for as long as possible.*

The ideal time for a facelift is usually at the onset of these wrinkles in the 40's, rather than after they have creased deeply into the face. A more limited operation, a cheeklift or *meloplasty*, can clear the jawline and lessen the jowls in most younger patients. However, when the degree of sagging is greater and more correction required, a full face and necklift *(rhytidectomy)* is required for complete treatment of temple, cheek and neck areas. In those with acne-scarred skin, the thickening, loss of tone and puffiness frequently result in an earlier need for facelifting.

In recommending that facelifts be performed sooner rather than later, I must emphasize that *there must be something to correct!* All surgery has some risk, and the "end-point", the desired result, must justify that risk. *Facelifts cannot be performed "prophylactically".*

A cheeklift, with or without eyelid lift, can be readily and safely performed in the office on most patients. As the extent of the operation increases into and beyond a full facelift—or in the presence of any medical problems—a short hospitalization is required. This is preferred, not so much for technical reasons, but *to minimize patient movement* during the first 24 to 36 hours.

By making incisions in front of and behind the ear, the skin of the face can be mobilized from the temple areas to the eyebrows, from the cheek bones to the cheeks, and to the folds at the corners of the mouth, and the neck totally. Pulling this skin taut in a backward and upward direction can remove most of these wrinkles that have accumulated with time. Scars are within the patient's hairline and are covered by the hair; if the procedure is performed well, it does not change the visage or expression of the face.

Customarily, *local anesthesia is preferable* because of its added safety and the advantage of patient cooperation. As true of most plastic surgical procedures, this is local anesthesia *supplemented with premedications and intravenous relaxants.* However, some patients prefer general anesthesia and *I prefer general anesthesia whenever the procedure requires extensive neck correction or surgery on deeper structures.*

CASE HISTORIES

N.L. was a 55-year-old housewife who had become a widow three years ago after a lengthy, emotionally-taxing bout with her husband's cancer. Her period of grieving was over and she wished to again become active in the charities and social events that had occupied her time and given purpose to her life before her husband's illness. Time and the hardship of the last few years, together with a rather marked weight loss, all had produced "an aging face". The creased-in wrinkles of the last few years were not happy ones. Deep hollows grooved her cheeks beneath pronounced eyelid bags and jowls squared her delicate jawline. Crepey, saggy neck skin kept her constantly in covering turtle-neck styles. Make-up from her chin usually wound up on her clothing.

Wishing to improve her appearance, she consulted me for a face and eyelid lift which I performed in the hospital under local anesthesia. Afterwards she again became meticulous about her appearance, picked out some new clothes and a new hairstyle and started to mingle with her former friends. During postoperative follow-up, I began to rely on her reviews of Broadway shows and new restaurants. There is no question that she was happier and very pleased that the procedure had been performed.

N.P. was a 54-year-old real estate broker married to a somewhat younger professional woman. Even though their marriage was very happy and secure, with two growing children, he felt that he looked very much older than his wife who was constantly meeting younger men in her work. The patient had his face and eyes done to remove the jowls, eyelid bags and crepey neck skin. He also had a small chin implant to strengthen his jawline and help clean up his neck. He was very pleased with the result, and his wife admitted afterwards that she had harbored similar thoughts—which she had kept to herself for fear of hurting her husband—and was very happy he had gone ahead with the surgery on his own.

PREPARATION

Professional photographs are required to help the surgeon plan his procedure and call to his attention particular problems which may require specific measures for correction. As for all elective surgery, *Vitamin E and aspirin-containing drugs are avoided for two weeks prior to surgery*, and *Vitamin K and Vitamin C are prescribed.*

If the surgery is to proceed in the office, preliminary blood tests are drawn during the preceding week. The patient should *not* come to surgery with a sunburn and peeling skin. *Skin care before surgery should be meticulous*, preferably according to the previously-discussed principles. Everything should be optimal for a good result.

Someone contemplating a facelift should set aside approximately two weeks and should expect to look rather bruised and swollen for the first week and a half, with the face being somewhat puffy and having several black and blue marks around the chin and neck. All sutures are removed by ten days and a general return to social life is possible in two weeks, although rarely some bruises may still have to be covered with make-up at this time.

It is wise to refrain from having one's hair bleached until all the scalp suture lines are well-healed at three weeks from surgery. Therefore, any regular hair bleaching or coloring should be done a few days before the scheduled surgery. If you are planning to lose any weight, it is preferable to do so *before* rather than after surgery.

The night before surgery, the patient showers and shampoos with *Phisohex®*. The patient should bring a pair of sunglasses and a scarf or hat to the office or hospital to wear on his or her way home. Shirts, blouses and sweaters that button in front will be more convenient than pull-over types.

THE PROCEDURE

If the patient is having local anesthesia, heavy premedication is employed and the patient is further sedated with intravenous relaxants while the hair is being sectioned and the surgical incisions planned. If general anesthesia is employed (this requires hospitalization), the patient is put to sleep before anything happens and will be totally unaware of anything which follows. Even under local anesthesia, patients usually have very little recall of the procedure and are in total comfort at all times.

For a full facelift, an S-shaped incision is planned several inches behind the hairline. It begins several inches above the ear in the temple area, continues in the crease between the ear and the side of the face, around the earlobe, behind the ear onto the back portion of the ear itself, and into the scalp behind the ear just above the level of the ear canal (see **Fig. 2**). The more neck correction required, the further I carry the incision behind the ear to the midline in back. For a cheeklift, the forward incision stops below the top of the ear. In men, the temple incision is placed somewhat further back so that it will never be seen, even if temple balding should occur.

The only portion of the incision near the face itself is the 2 1/4 inches in front of the ear. This area heals very inconspicuously; it is a natural facial crease. Sutures are removed very early, and one is hard-pressed to see it by as early as two weeks. I prefer to dart the incision above and below the little cartilaginous prominence in front of the ear canal (the *tragus*) because of the tendency for incisions placed behind it to open up the ear canal unattractively to view. I draw lines from the ears to the eyes, nose and mouth on both sides of the face to guarantee symmetry in lifting.

Beginning on the right side, the skin around the ear is first numbed with injections of local anesthetic through a very fine-gauge needle. Then the skin of the temple, cheek and neck is numbed with a longer needle inserted through the area that has been already numbed. The anesthetic has *epinephrine* in it to minimize bleeding and for this reason is used even when the procedure is performed under general anesthesia.

After skin of the face has been anesthetized, the incisions are made and the skin is freed from its underlying attachments by blunt spreading with scissors. All tiny bleeders are then sealed with electrocautery. (Any cheek augmentation, fat, fascia or muscle corrections are done at this time.)

The skin of the face and neck is then lifted in an upwards and backward direction. Pilot sutures are placed for alignment above and below the ear. Care is taken not to move the sideburn too far upwards. In men, some beard-bearing skin may be brought behind the earlobe and later require either daily shaving or electrolysis. Care is taken not to cause irregularity in the hairline behind the ear so that the hair may be worn "up" in women and so that this presents no problem for men with shorter hair.

The scalp incisions are closed with individual sutures. The suture lines in front of and behind the ear are closed with fine continuous sutures. Soft, flat drains are placed in the scalp incisions above and behind the ear to allow any oozing to collect on the dressing rather than beneath the skin. The procedure is then repeated on the other side.

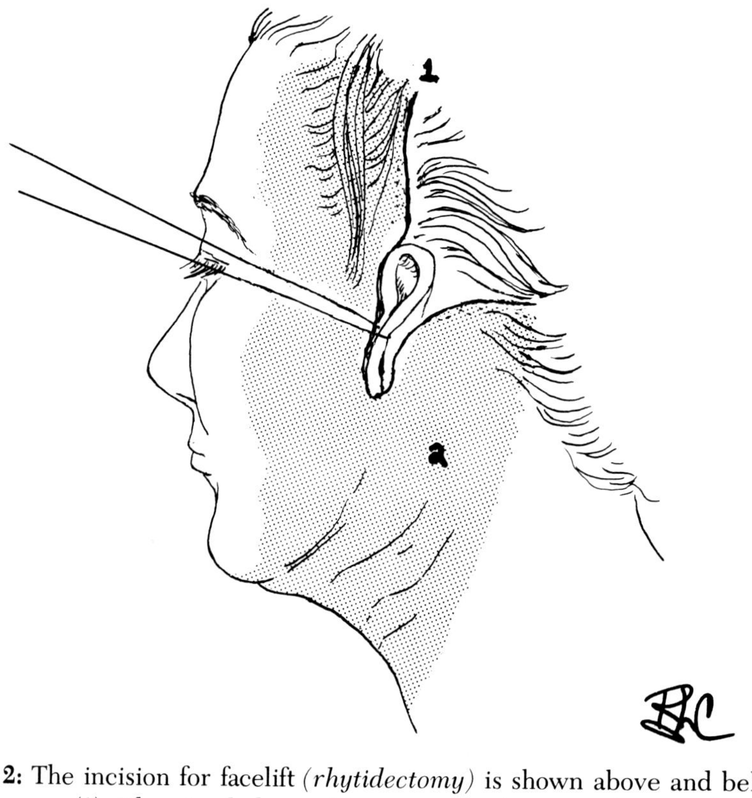

FIGURE 2: The incision for facelift *(rhytidectomy)* is shown above and behind the ear (1). The stippled area (2) represents the area of surgicial undermining. (Reprinted from *The Kindest Cut*.)

If the eyelid lifting is to be done at the time of facelifting, as it frequently is, I always do the face before I do the lower lids. Slightly more lower eyelid skin can be removed after the facelift.

Sometimes a little redundant skin still remains on the neck; in this case, after injection with local anesthesic, a small, curved incision is made in the shadow line beneath the chin to allow removal of additional skin (and fat) in this area. This same incision allows access to the muscles beneath if correction of neck bands requires it. This incision is closed with fine interrupted sutures. I can usually anticipate the need for this incision preoperatively.

A bulky dressing is then placed on the face and neck consisting of molded cotton and wrap-around bandages. It looks something like a roller derby helmut and is deliberately tight. It is critical in minimizing bruising and will be kept in place for 24 to 36 hours postoperatively.

RECUPERATION

You will lie flat on your back with a folded sheet beneath your shoulders for the first night. You will have no pain, but the dressing will be uncomfortable. Keeping your head back and your neck extended without a pillow makes the "chin-strap" portion of the dressing much less binding. *Chewing, talking, and much walking are discouraged on the day of surgery.* Therefore, I recommend against bedside telephones and visitors the night of surgery and the following day.

The bulky dressing and drains will be removed the following day and replaced with a much lighter "turban" dressing. You will then be allowed to return home if the procedure was performed in the hospital. A scarf or cap can cover the dressing. If an eyelid lift was performed concurrently, sunglasses can be used to cover your eyes. A few hospitalized patients prefer to remain an additional day so that all eyelid sutures may be removed before they return home.

The sutures in front of the ear are removed on the 5th day, those behind the ear on the 7th and all scalp sutures on the 10th day. You may shampoo on the 5th day (again with *Phisohex®*), towel-dry your hair, and gently brush it. Almost all bruising will be gone by the end of the second week. Any small, residual black-and-blue marks can be covered with make-up, and you may appear socially at this time.

When this procedure is performed on someone in his or her late 60's, the patient must be informed that a small touch-up may be necessary fairly soon (6 months to a year) after the initial procedure to obtain the optimal result. This is because, at this age, the skin lacks the elasticity of that of the younger patient, with whom the surgeon can achieve a longer (5–10 year) response to the facelift. This loss of elasticity is also found in markedly sun-damaged skin.

Jowls are lessened by the procedure but are not completely eliminated. This is because the branches of the facial nerve limit the surgery that can be done in this region. This is one of the reasons why it is preferable to intercede surgically before jowls are well-developed. *Facelifting can turn back the clock and perhaps slow it down, but surgery can't stop it.*

Smile lines are not totally eliminated by facelifting. Indeed, *a smile is one wrinkle that should never be removed!* I will not perform a facelift on a patient who desires an artificially tight and pulled look. I would be ashamed to acknowledge the shiny skin, the unnaturally wide mouth, and flaring nostrils of such a patient as being of my creation. A typical result of a cheek and necklift is shown in **Photos 3** and **4**.

PRECAUTIONS AND POTENTIAL PROBLEMS

A *temporary numbness* of the earlobes may persist for several weeks. During this time, it is wise to either refrain from wearing earrings or to keep track of wearing time to prevent damage to the earlobes. Sections of the scalp are also often temporarily anesthetized. Therefore, the lowest setting on hair dryers and blowers should be used to prevent unfelt burns to the scalp. These effects gradually resolve within several weeks.

A collection of blood or serum, termed a *hematoma*, may accumulate beneath the facial skin, a complication that occurs 3–5% of the time in most surgeons' hands. However, when it does occur, removal of the fluid is usually possible without a return to the operating room, if the amount of fluid is not excessively large. Usually the only difference noted by the patient with this complication may be a temporary increase in black-and-blue bruising over the neck and jaw.

Rarely, surgery may result in *injury to a branch of the facial nerve* to the mouth or forehead. Almost all of these injuries are of only a temporary nature and resolve in several weeks.

Rarely again, if sufficient undermining was carried out, a scalp *scar* may spread and be objectionable. Should it be required, scars can be easily revised in the office under local anesthesia. *Hair loss* should not occur if undermining was carried out at the proper level. However, should this occur, any bald area is usually amenable to office treatment.

Skin care after surgery should be meticulous. Hypoallergenic make-up may be gently applied to the face in all areas except suture lines by the 5th day and even to suture lines at 10 days. It should be *gently and completely removed at night with a soapless cleanser.* A *gentle clarifier* should be incorporated into the postoperative regimen and a *moisturizer with Vitamin E* is particularly helpful in healing. All skin manipulation should be in a *gentle, upwards direction.* Exposure to extremes of heat or cold should be avoided in the immediate postoperative period.

Prolonged exposure to direct sunlight should be avoided for 3 to 6 weeks. If this is unavoidable, a *SPF 12-15 sunblock with PABA* should be employed. After the 6 weeks, *SPF 6-9 sunscreens* provide adequate protection.

FINISHING TOUCHES

I usually *remove any warts, moles or spiders* at the time of facelifting or in the immediate postoperative visits. I also lightly *dermabrade any age spots* that have not responded to previous treatment with a *hydroquinone* fade cream.

The eyelids often require corrective *blepharoplasty* at the time of cheek or facelifting. Otherwise, the eyelid bags become more noticeable because of their contrast with the rest of the face.

As discussed in previous chapters, the finer wrinkles which are not eliminated by facelifting may be removed through applications of a *chemical peel.* A chemical peel may be performed at the time of facelifting but is more commonly performed as a separate office procedure to avoid jeopardy to undermined skin. However, if only fine wrinkles about the mouth are a problem, the "muzzle area" of the face—the upper and lower lips, and the chin between laughlines—may be peeled at the time of facelift *(perioral peel).* A full-face peel is scheduled at least 3 weeks after the facelift. *Collagen injections* may also be employed to remove any isolated fine wrinkles remaining after surgery.

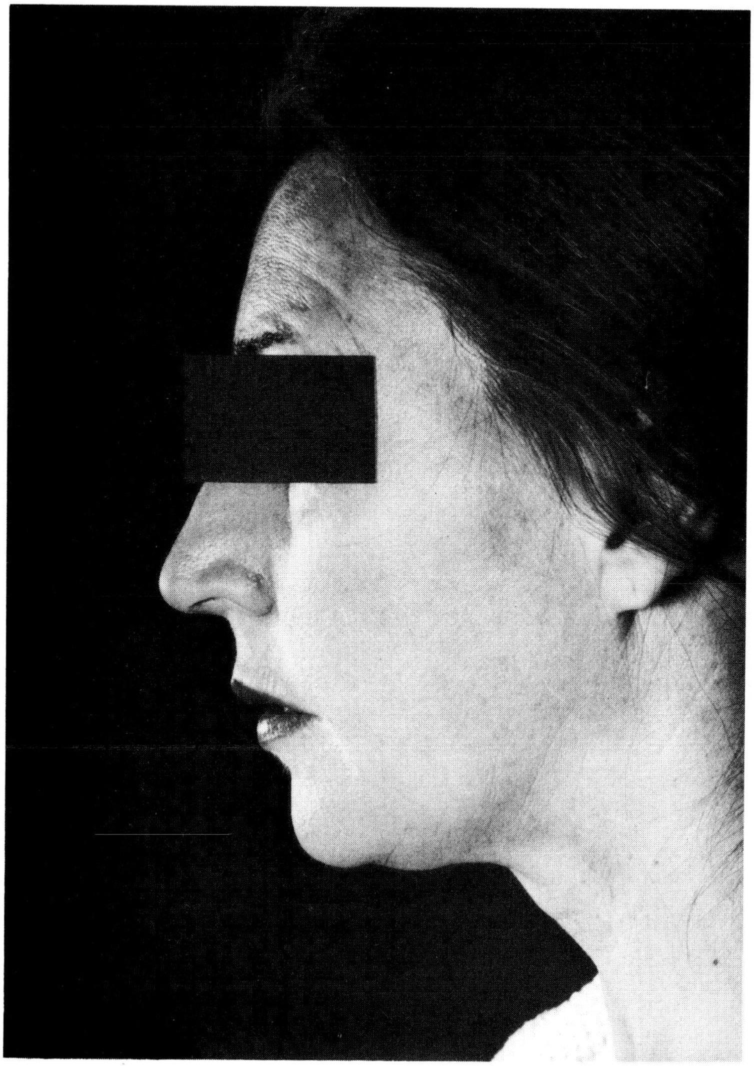

PHOTO 3: A patient with early jowling obscuring neck and jawline.

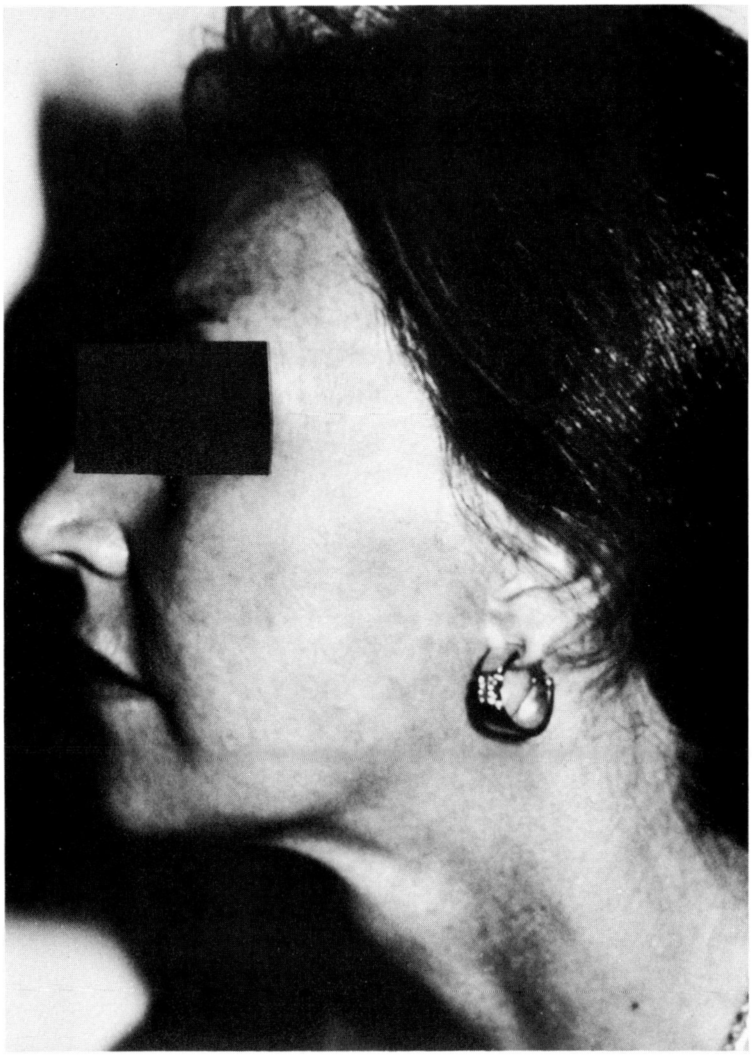

PHOTO 4: The same patient after cheek and necklift.

In a young person, the angle of the jaw is sharp and clean without double or triple chins. Frequently, an excision of redundant skin and fat locally, in the offending area beneath the chin, is helpful in smoothing out the neck beyond what can be attained by a facelift alone. The surgeon should inform patients when this additional procedure will be necessary. This "chin tuck" is called a *submental lipectomy* and, if not performed with the facelift, may be done subsequently in the office on an outpatient basis. This surgery does result in a hairline scar beneath the chin but it is in an area which is not readily noticeable.

Although a facelift and a submental tuck may still result in marked improvements, patients with low *hyoid* bones (the bones at the root of the tongue) will *not* have a completely sharp angle between the throat and chin no matter what technique is used. Sometimes adding prominence to the chin with an *augmentation mentoplasty* may result in further improvement.

With aging, facial subcutaneous fat decreases and cheek bones and chins frequently appear less prominent. The high cheek bone effect so desireable to many patients can be obtained by prosthetic implants. Such *cheek augmentation* may be done after a facelift to enhance the operative result. *Chin augmentation* may be done through the mouth or through the incision beneath the chin if a submental lipectomy is done. Both procedures may result in a striking improvement of appearance in well-chosen patients and do not significantly lengthen the facelift procedure or alter the patient's postoperative care.

Although our body growth stops with adulthood, earlobes continue to grow and noses tend to droop. These are subtle signs of aging. *Earlobes may be made smaller* and more youthful, and *plunging nasal tips may be lifted* at the time of facelift with little lengthening of the surgical procedure and no additional time required for convalescence.

Similarly, the upper-third of the face may require direct attention with a forehead lift performed concurrently at the time of facelifting. Sagging eyebrows can be lifted, forehead wrinkles and creases at the root of the nose can be lessened, and scowl lines eliminated by this means.

Some balding men may choose to follow a facelift with hair transplants. Occasionally, portions of the scalp to be removed during the procedure may even be suitable for hair plug donors which can be placed at that time.

Chemical peels and eyelid lifts were discussed in previous chapters; all of the other "finishing touches" mentioned above are fully described in the sections which follow . . .

CHAPTER 11

Raising Sagging Brows

The top one-third of the face is not exempt from the aging process. In fact, time frequently stamps the forehead with its signature long before it affects the rest of the face. Horizontal wrinkles first crease the brow only during expression. Then, they soon take up permanent residence. Arching wrinkles may form several tiers above the outer eyebrows. Quite often these wrinkles are not symmetric but are more accentuated on one side of the face than the other. Vertical furrows may separate the eyebrows and remain as constant "scowl" lines to give a stern expression to the face.

The eyebrows seldom stay perched on the eye socket rims, but gradually descend. Women have know this for generations as mothers have taught their daughters how to pluck their eyebrows and use eyebrow pencils appropriately. Much of the redundant upper eyelid skin which develops is caused by eyebrow droop. As the forehead sags as a unit, horizontal creases form at the root of the nose and the temple area pleats into crow's feet radiating from the corners of the eyes.

The squinting associated with bright outdoor sun, uncorrected poor vision, habitual reading in poor light, and perhaps even uncomfortable or poorly-fitting contacts, causes the circular muscle about the eyelids *(orbicularis oculi)* to exert its strength to force the brow to droop and create crow's feet.

Fortunately, the situation is readily correctable and the eyebrows may be returned to their proper positions by two methods. The first method, a *direct eyebrow lift*, I perform *very rarely* because surgeon and patient must depend upon a facial scar healing perfectly—a risk I prefer to take only when necessary.

An ellipse of skin is removed immediately above the eyelids and the eyelids are brought directly to their former location. The procedure is minor, may be readily performed under local anesthesia in the office, and sutures are removed in 5 to 7 days. However, the scar is in a visible location and I am loath to perform this procedure *unless:*

(1) the patient is a somewhat older individual in whom scars will blanch sooner and blend into existing wrinkles easier;

(2) the patient is fair-skinned enough to permit dermabrasion to be carried out should the scar prove objectionable;

(3) the patient is a woman willing to cover any traces of scar with an eyebrow pencil;

(4) the patient has a high forehead which would only be rendered higher by a forehead lift as described below.

The second procedure, which I much prefer, is a forehead or *coronal lift.* An incision is made from the top of one ear to the other about three inches behind the hairline. I prefer to avoid this procedure in men whose families have a history of balding. Even in suitable candidates, the incision must be far back enough so that, if male-pattern balding occurs, the scars will not be exposed.

The scalp is lifted from its attachments, the sagging brow is lifted, restored to proper location, and redundant scalp excised. Generally, to enhance and prolong the result, the muscles which cause scowl lines are deliberately rendered ineffectual as are the muscles which wrinkle the brow.

The procedure may be readily carried out in the office under local anesthesia and all sutures are removed by the 10th day. If hospitalization is selected for medical reasons or those of convenience, only an overnight stay is customary. Two weeks need be set aside for the procedure since there may be substantial temporary swelling and bruising, generally about the eyelids. Since a forehead lift is frequently done in conjunction with eyelid surgery, it is well to note that the forehead lift should *precede* eyelid surgery since less redundant upper eyelid skin will remain after the procedure.

CASE HISTORIES

Although a forehead lift is so frequently performed with facelifting that it is difficult to provide an example of it as a solitary procedure, I believe the patient described below well illustrates its indications.

M.L. was a 34-year-old legal secretary whose sensitive eyelids had been intermittently swollen for as long as she could remember. She had frequently used mineral oil-based eyelid moisturizers and loved the beaches. She was concerned that she had a low forehead and that her droopy eyebrows combined with her puffy eyelids to give her a very sleepy-eyed and not-particularly-bright appearance. She wanted something to be done to "open up" and "wake-up" her seemingly small eyes.

Under local anesthesia, a concurrent forehead and upper eyelid lift was performed in the office. As will be discussed later, a hereditary deposit of fat was removed from the outer, upper eyelid and the prominent, down-sloping ridge of the outer eye socket—which gave her eye a downcast look—was removed. Afterwards, she was very pleased at her higher forehead and how much time she saved in the morning applying her eye make-up.

Although one of the lawyers in the firm did ask her out to dinner afterwards, to preserve the result achieved, she was cautioned to wear sunglasses at the beach to avoid squinting and to avoid mineral oil-based eyelid moisturizers.

PREPARATION

As is usual for cosmetic surgery, the patient should *avoid Vitamin E and aspirin-containing drugs for two weeks prior to surgery*, and *Vitamin C and Vitamin K are prescribed*. Again, *preoperative skin care should be meticulous* since no prudent surgeon would operate through a field of pimples or pustules electively. The patient will shampoo and shower with *Phisohex®* before surgery and wear *no make-up, false eyelashes, or contacts* on that day.

Any hair bleaching or coloring should be done several days prior to surgery so that fresh roots will not be visible during the first three weeks after surgery when it should be avoided.

Professional medical photographs and the usual *preliminary blood tests* are performed prior to surgery. Unless the forehead lift is to be performed in conjunction with other procedures, *local anesthesia is usually preferable* for its safety and the advantage of having patient cooperation. Hospitalization is only required for medical problems, extended procedures, patient preference, or for general anesthesia.

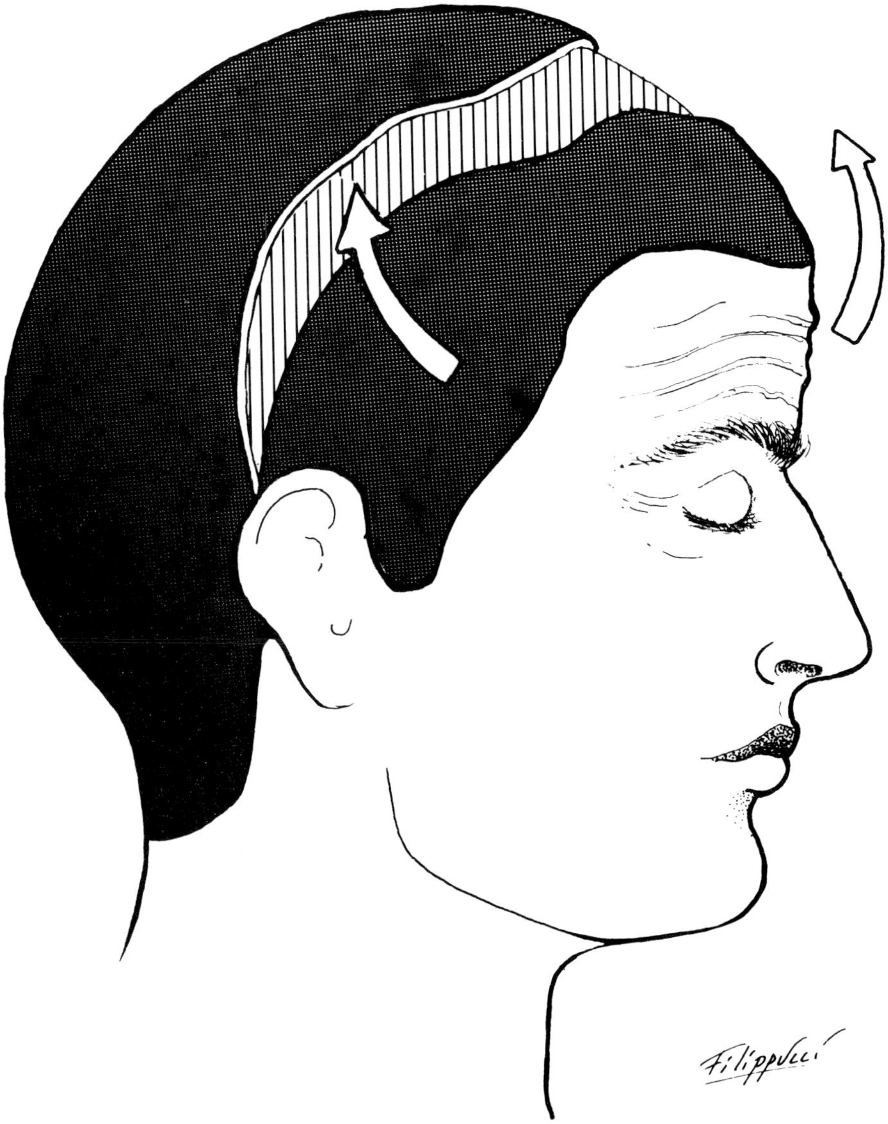

FIGURE 3: The scalp incision for raising sagging eyebrows and eliminating forehead wrinkles with a forehead *(coronal)* lift is shown and the arrows illustrate the direction of pull.

THE PROCEDURE

After the preoperative sedative injections have taken effect, the patient will be brought to the Operating Room where an intravenous will be started as a route of administration for further relaxants.

The hair will be sectioned and an incision planned about 3″ behind the hairline curving from above one ear to the other. The "mosquitoes" will bite as the site of the incision is numbed by injections of local anesthetic through a fine-gauge needle. A longer needle, placed through this previously-numbed area, will numb the rest of the forehead.

An incision is made through all layers of the scalp, and it is elevated down to the eyebrows (see **Fig. 3**). The upper portion of the circular muscle surrounding the eyes *(orbicularis oculi)* is lifted along with the forehead muscle *(frontalis)* so that the eyebrows may be raised to their proper places. Usually the muscles causing scowl lines *(corrugators)* are divided or excised and a strip of *frontalis* (which causes brow wrinkling) excised to prolong and enhance the result.

Pilot sutures are placed for alignment as I make sure the eyes close completely and comfortably. The procedure is *so* effective at removing upper lid redundancy caused by eyebrow sagging or *ptosis* that a surgeon can remove too much *if* he is not attentive to this detail. The underlying tissue is reapproximated with individual sutures of absorbable material. Then the scalp is closed with interrupted sutures—I like blue ones so I can see them easily to take them out!

A bulky dressing of molded cotton and wrap-around bandages, similar to that used in facelifting, is used and will remain in place for 24 hours.

RECUPERATION

The dressing will be removed on the following day and a light "turban" dressing be applied. Hospitalized patients may return home at this time with a scarf or cap to cover the dressing and tinted glasses to cover any bruising. You may shampoo after the 5th day (with *Phisohex*®) and all sutures are removed by the 10th day. Any mild shampoo may be used thereafter. The hair may again be bleached, colored, or receive a permanent 3 weeks after surgery.

Significant forehead and eyelid swelling usually occurs and the eyelids frequently bruise as well. Almost all bruising and swelling subsides by the second week and a little make-up can conceal any discolorations that remain.

Direct sun should be avoided for 3–6 weeks unless a *SPF 9-12 sunblock* is employed because it will increase and prolong any postoperative swelling. Afterwards, the routinely recommended *SPF 6-9 sunscreen* provides sufficient protection.

PRECAUTIONS AND POTENTIAL PROBLEMS

Portions of the scalp may be temporarily anesthetic after surgery. The lowest settings on hair driers and blowers should be used to avoid unfelt burns to the scalp. Electric rollers should be avoided until sensation returns over the next few weeks.

Rarely, as in facelifting, a collection of blood may occur (a *hematoma*) which requires removal, usually non-operative. If this occurs, it does not compromise the result, but only results in a temporary increase in the amount of bruising.

Rarely, if the underlying tissue was well-sewn, a *scalp scar* may spread and be objectionable. Should this occur, it can easily be revised in the office under local anesthesia.

FINISHING TOUCHES

Forehead lifts are frequently performed together with *eyelid lifts.* A not infrequent combination is the lower lids and forehead lift together. If the upper eyelid skin redundancy is mild and there is no associated fat, forehead lift alone may fully eliminate the problem.

A nice side effect of the forehead lift—that may be deliberately exploited by undermining to the very tip of the nose—is the slight lifting of a droopy nasal tip. A nasal tip refinement or *soft tissue rhinoplasty* may be carried out concurrently to enhance this effect.

If the middle third of the face is narrow and long compared to the forehead and lower face, as the forehead is raised with a forehead lift, the cheeks may be augmented with solid silicon implants inserted through the mouth to add width to the mid-face and improve the facial proportions. This adds little time to the surgical procedure and does not lengthen the convalescence.

It should be mentioned that bushy eyebrows are frequently associated with aging, particularly in men. Clipping the eyebrows slightly shorter may enhance the surgical rejunvenation in these patients.

Eyelid lifts for skin redundancy have been discussed previously; their modifications to include bony expansion, as well as nasal reprofiling and cheek augmentation are fully described in future chapters . . .

* * *

CHAPTER 12

Lipshaping

The mouth is extremely expressive and communicates our emotions as much and sometimes more than our eyes. Happiness, sadness and tension all are conveyed by the mouth. There is no more flattering feature on the face than a smile; a pleasing pair of lips in front of nice teeth can turn a dull face into an inviting one.

In women particularly, a fuller pair of lips carries a sensuous connotation. Thin lips appear more harsh and stern. The lips frequently become thinner with aging; this is one of the reasons for the development of the fine wrinkles which radiate from the mouth in old age. Lipstick and lip-liners can make up in part for a deficiency, but only partly, because they cannot add substance to a thin lip, but only simulate more *vermilion*, the colored portion of the lips.

Many men and women of some races may consider themselves too well endowed in the lip department. For them, the desire is to reduce the bulk and size of lips that seem out of proportion to the rest of the face.

Lip surgery or *cheiloplasty* is a fairly simple office procedure, performed under local anesthesia, that can yield dramatic results. To make the lips fuller, tissue is shifted from the inside towards the outside; to thin the lips tissue is removed on the inside. All incisions are within the mouth so that nothing but the result shows outside. The effect in well-chosen patients can be quite dramatic.

CASE HISTORIES

P.G. was a 42-year-old housewife who had always considered herself rather "sexless". To compensate for this, she made it a point to excell in athletics and had developed a very good tennis and golf game. Her lips were very thin, and although she used lipstick well to camouflage this defect, she had always longed for a fuller, more sensuous pair of lips. She always felt that her lips disappeared from view when she smiled and was self-conscious about it.

In the office, under local anesthesia, inside lining was shifted to make her upper lip fuller. Afterwards, she was so pleased with the result that she felt her smile was now an asset. She had two of her front teeth "bonded" to complete the picture and then allowed her family to photograph her smiling!

G.W. was a 26-year-old black model who felt that her rather thick lips spoiled her otherwise very striking face. She even had a rather strange maneuver down pat in which she flattened her lips for photographs by slightly pursing them. She wished something be done to thin them permanently.

In the office, under local anesthesia, both upper and lower lips were thinned. Even before the postoperative swelling subsided, she had some photographs taken and didn't even have to use her "special maneuver" to get the look she wanted.

PREPARATION

As usual, *professional medical photographs* are required to illustrate the patient's precise needs. *Aspirin and aspirin-containing products should be avoided for two weeks before surgery* and *Vitamin K and Vitamin C are prescribed* to minimize bruising.

On the morning of surgery, you should wash your face with *Phisohex®* to eliminate any troublesome bacteria. You should brush your teeth and rinse your mouth out with hydrogen peroxide and Listerine® before coming to the office. Wear *no lipstick, lip-liner or make-up* on that day.

Set aside approximately a week for the procedure. Bruising is minimal, but the swelling usually takes 4–6 days to subside.

THE PROCEDURE

After you have received premedicating injections and intravenous relaxants, your lips are numbed with injections of location anesthetic.

If the lips are to be made fuller *(augmentation cheiloplasty)*, several V-shaped incisions, generally three per lip, are made on the *mucosa* (lining of the mouth) inside the mouth with top of the V facing the lips, slightly turned towards the center. These "tongues" or *flaps* of tissue are undermined and shifted towards the outside. The V incision is then closed in the pattern of a Y. This is the basic *V-Y plasty* of plastic surgery which has a multitude of other applications.

If the lips are to be made thinner *(reduction cheiloplasty)*, ellipses are drawn for excision parallel to the borders of the lips on the inside. I estimate their width by gently pinching the *mucosa* with specially-made blunt tweezers. After injection of local anesthetic, the *mucosa* within these ellipses is removed. If necessary, a portion of the muscle beneath which surrounds the lips *(orbicularis oris)* is removed as well.

In both cases, any bleeding is controlled with electrocautery and incisions are closed with absorbable sutures so that no removal is necessary.

RECUPERATION

There is usually very little bruising, but the lips usually swell considerably, and this swelling may persist for several days. Ice packs to the lips for the first 24 hours can substantially reduce this swelling.

The patient takes a *fluid diet that evening* and a *soft diet* that requires little chewing *for the following day*. The mouth is rinsed with a mixture of salt water and hydrogen peroxide after eating for the first few days. I prefer that the patient does not smoke for the first 24 hours if it is at all possible. This is a good time to quit!

No kissing is allowed for four days and the front teeth should be brushed *gently*. At the end of a week's time, the patient is ready to be seen socially.

PRECAUTIONS AND POTENTIAL COMPLICATIONS

Poor planning, technical error on the part of the surgeon, or the vagaries of wound healing may result in the *possible need for a small subsequent revision* to obtain perfect symmetry or augmentation of the initial result achieved.

Although the mucosa usually heals quite well, a firmness or *hypertrophic scar* may result in some Blacks and require several injections of *Kenalog®* to cause its resolution. This is a steroid capable of causing the softening of *hypertrophic* scars or their more exuberant relatives, termed *keloids*.

FINISHING TOUCHES

If there are multiple fine wrinkles surrounding and radiating from the lips, these may respond to perioral peel, dermabrasion or collagen injections. For one or two solitary wrinkles, I prefer *collagen injections*. The wrinkle itself is treated and the slightly-raised "white roll", which surrounds the vermilion, is "beefed up" as well, since its disappearance is partly responsible for the development of the wrinkle.

For many or multiple wrinkles about the mouth, I perform a *perioral* or "muzzle area" *dermabrasion*—including the lips, chin and the area beneath the nose and between the laughlines—followed by application of a *Hydron®* dressing to alleviate any postoperative discomfort and accelerate healing.

For those with a moderate number of wrinkles about the mouth and with very fair complexions, I prefer a *perioral peel*. The technical advantages and disadvantages of each procedure for a particular patient's problem and complexion govern my choice.

If the lips are being thinned, the nose can be narrowed and height added to the bridge in a *rhinoplasty* in patients desiring an enhancement of this effect.

Any *dental restoration* planned can obviously complete the picture of a pleasing smile. The newer "bonding" many dentists are carrying out can achieve dramatic results in proper patients.

Dermabrasions, chemical peels and collagen injections have been described previously. Nasal reprofiling and *rhinoplasty* to correct ethnic traits will be discussed in a future chapter . . .

* * *

PART II
FACEMAKING

A. Fat Contouring

CHAPTER 13

Eliminating Eyelid Bags

In many patients, there is more than redundant skin causing the appearance of a tired and aging eye. The eye socket is filled with fat which cushions the eye with every step. However, with time, some of this fat protrudes from its proper location and causes eyelid pouches or bags to form. In the upper lid, this fat is most frequently above the inner portion and towards the outer portion of the eyelid. In the lower eyelid, the fat is most commonly all the way across. Since the cheek skin is attached to the bottom rim of the eye socket, the lower eyelid bag is accentuated by the hollow which develops immediately beneath it.

In some young patients, who develop upper eyelid bags in their early 20's, there may be a separate pocket of fat towards the outer portion of the eyelid, quite distinct from those protruding from about the eye, which is present and responsible for the upper eyelid fullness. This frequently is a familial trait.

Removing the fat associated with these bags has a remarkably rejuvenating effect which restores a well-rested look to the eye. On rare occasions, there may be *only* offending fat. In these cases, the lower eyelid fat can be removed *transconjunctivally*, that is without a skin incision. However, much more commonly there is an associated redundancy of skin which requires the *blepharoplasty* approach described previously. Removal of the upper eyelid fat which causes a fullness and droopiness of the lid, tends to "open" up the eye because it allows the eyelid fold to be more clearly seen.

In Oriental patients, there is another location for the fat, *between* the muscle which lifts the eyelid *(levator tarsi superioris)* and the skin. If the

Oriental lid or "single eye" is to be "Westernized", this fat pocket must be eliminated before surgery can be performed on the muscle beneath to establish a "double eye".

In preliminary examination of the patient and in careful review of the preoperative photographs, I make note of the amount and location of any offending fat. When performing the surgery, I first remove the redundant skin as described previously and then explore the locations in which I have previously noted the presence of protruding fat. Fat removal adds no additional time to the convalescence, still permits local anesthesia and office surgery, and, when indicated, greatly improves the result.

CASE HISTORY

M.N. was a 28-year-old airline stewardess who had always been troubled by upper eyelid bags as had her mother at the same age. She frequently received on-the-job comments such as "And what did you do last night, Sweetheart?" She wanted something to be done to improve the situation.

Under local anesthesia in the office, the fat and a small amount of extra skin were removed from her upper lids. The patient was very pleased with her rested and awake look. Although the comments afterwards were still tasteless, they were more of the order of "What are you doing tonight, Honey?" and therefore somewhat more tolerable.

She was cautioned about the drying effects of a smoke-filled airplane at high altitudes and the necessity of eyelid moisturizing to preserve her good result.

PREPARATION

The preparation is identical to that previously described for *blepharoplasty*. Especially important are *quality, close-up, medical photographs in an upright position* to illustrate the location and amount of protruding fat.

PROCEDURE

Access is obtained by the *blepharoplasty* incisions described previously. There are generally two separate fat pockets in the upper lid and three in the lower in addition to the locations for familial and ethnic fat mentioned above.

In each area, the circular eyelid muscle *(orbicularis oculi)* is gently spread (or a strip excised if an eyelid festoon is present) and the individual fat pocket entered. Fat is allowed to herniate with gentle pressure upon the upper eyelid and underlying eye (see **Fig. 4**). After injection of local anesthesic, a clamp is placed upon the base of this extra fat and the protruding portion is excised. Light cautery upon this clamp seals any small bleeding sites. *Only so much fat is excised as is required to remove the eyelid bag.* The fat is sculpted to achieve a perfectly flat, non-pouchy lid.

After any indicated procedures upon the muscle or bone are performed, the incisions are sewn as previously described for eyelid lifts.

RECUPERATION

The convalescence is as for routine eyelid lifting with sutures being removed by the 3rd or 4th day. Bruising usually resolves by the end of the second week.

PRECAUTIONS AND POTENTIAL PROBLEMS

Bleeding or *hematoma* can occur rarely but if recognized and treated promptly, can usually be evacuated with little consequence to the patient except a little more than average bruising.

If the surgeon has been over-zealous in removing fat, the eye can attain a sunken appearance. This should not occur if care is taken, but if it does, it can be corrected by free fat grafts.

FINISHING TOUCHES

Many patients, particularly young ones and those with the habit of squinting, may have overly-developed eyelid muscles which cause unattractive eyelid *festoons.* In these patients, the offending muscle must be excised.

In some patients, *crow's feet* are particularly pronounced. These may be alleviated by partly dividing and spreading out the circular muscle which causes them at the corner of the eye. If forehead sag augments this effect, a forehead lift, which has been described previously, or a *temporal tuck* may further improve this problem. A temporal tuck is *not a minilift* but is the top portion of a facelift *with undermining* which affects the cheek, temple and outer brow area.

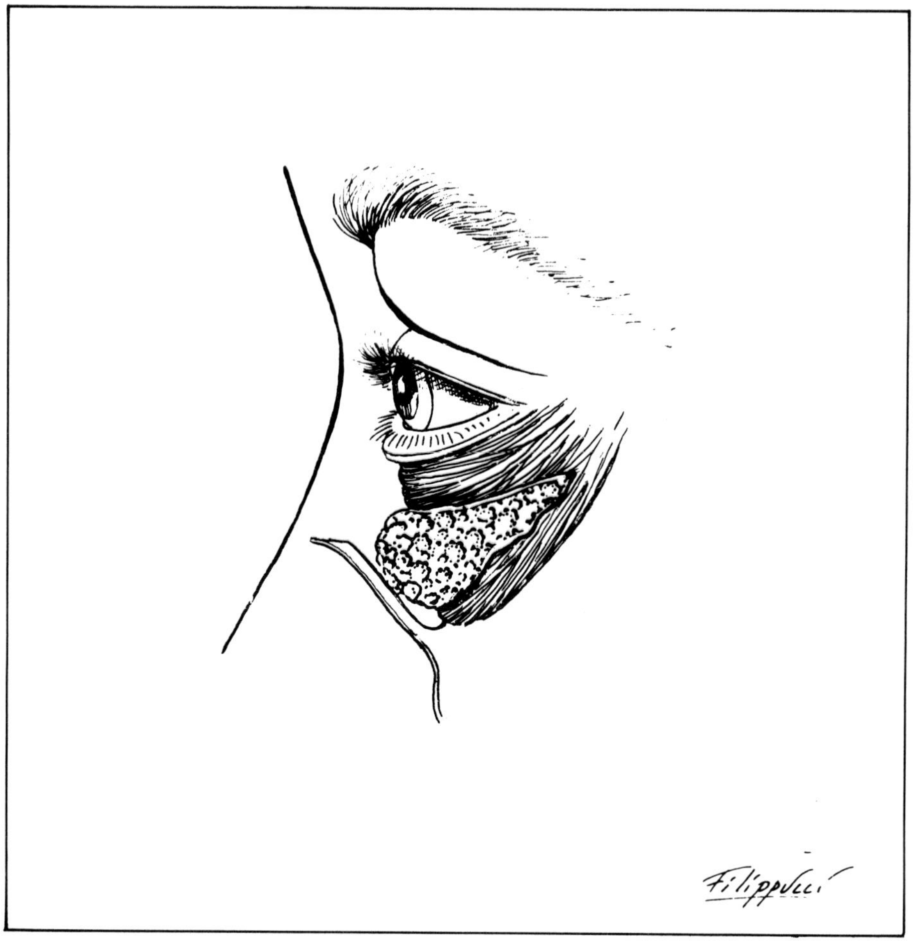

FIGURE 4: After the *orbital septum* is incised, the fat responsible for an eyelid bag protrudes between the separated fibers of eyelid muscle.

If the hollow under the eyelid bag *(nasojugal fold)* is particularly well-pronounced and offensive, I occasionally will use a portion of fat from the inner fat pocket to bolster or fill in this depression at the time of *blepharoplasty* (see **Photos 5** and **6**). A cheeklift or *meloplasty* may also help by restoring the thicker, sagging cheek skin to its proper location with elimination of the dimpling caused by its tethering to the eye socket rim. Simultaneous *cheek augmentation*, when indicated, can also help remove these unattractive valleys.

If the upper, outer eye socket rim is unduly prominent or sloping and covers the outer portion of the upper eyelid, making the eye appear smaller and "sadder", this projecting bone may be shaved away to achieve a more open, "happier" eye.

Surgery for redundant eyelid skin has been discussed previously and procedures on the eyelid muscles, the oriental eye, bony eye socket, and cheek bones are described in the chapters which follow . . .

* * *

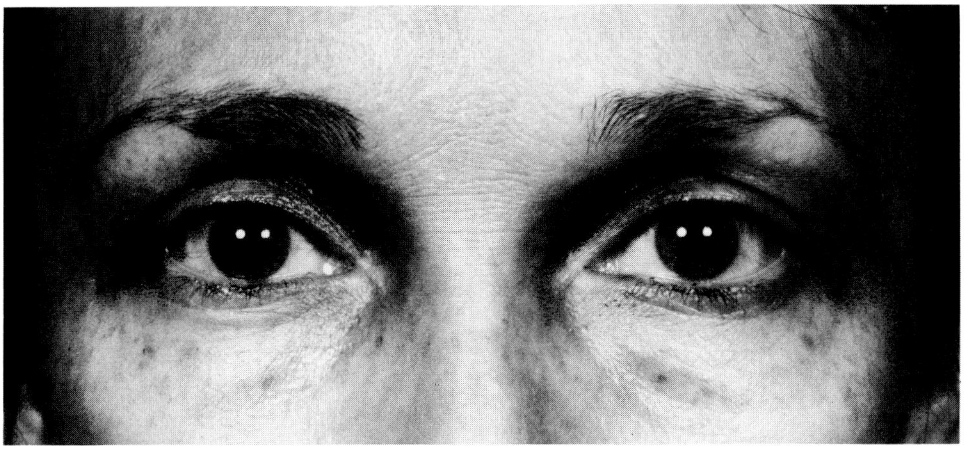

PHOTO 5: A patient with redundant skin of her upper and lower lids, dark circles below lower lids and marked *nasojugal folds* (cheek hollows beneath the lower lids).

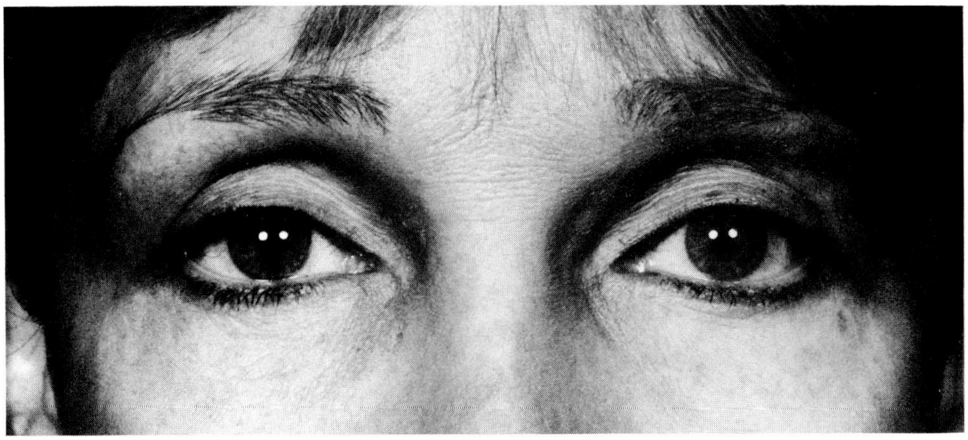

PHOTO 6: The same patient after eyelid lift.

CHAPTER 14

Removal of Under-the-Chin Fat

Many young people are plagued by familial deposits of fat under the chin. As they get older, this very much emphasizes any neck wrinkling and may form unattractive double or even triple chins. Weight reduction frequently has no effect upon this localized problem. In older patients, even after a face and necklift, there may be a residual deposit of offensive fat beneath the chin which detracts from an otherwise pleasing result. In both of these categories of patients, a localized assault on the problem area may be indicated.

A curved incision may be made in the shadow line beneath the chin and the extra fat trimmed away and sculpted for a clean neckline. When needed, a chin implant may be placed and if vertical neck bands are present, the *platysmal bands* causing the problem may be simultaneously treated. When the incision is closed, any redundant skin may be removed as well. The procedure is amenable to office surgery under local anesthesia.

In those with "pointy" chins, a specially-sculpted chin implant may be placed and the skin removal so planned as to give a more rounded chin and jawline. Sutures are removed within 7 days, bruising is usually minimal, and only a week need be set aside for the procedure.

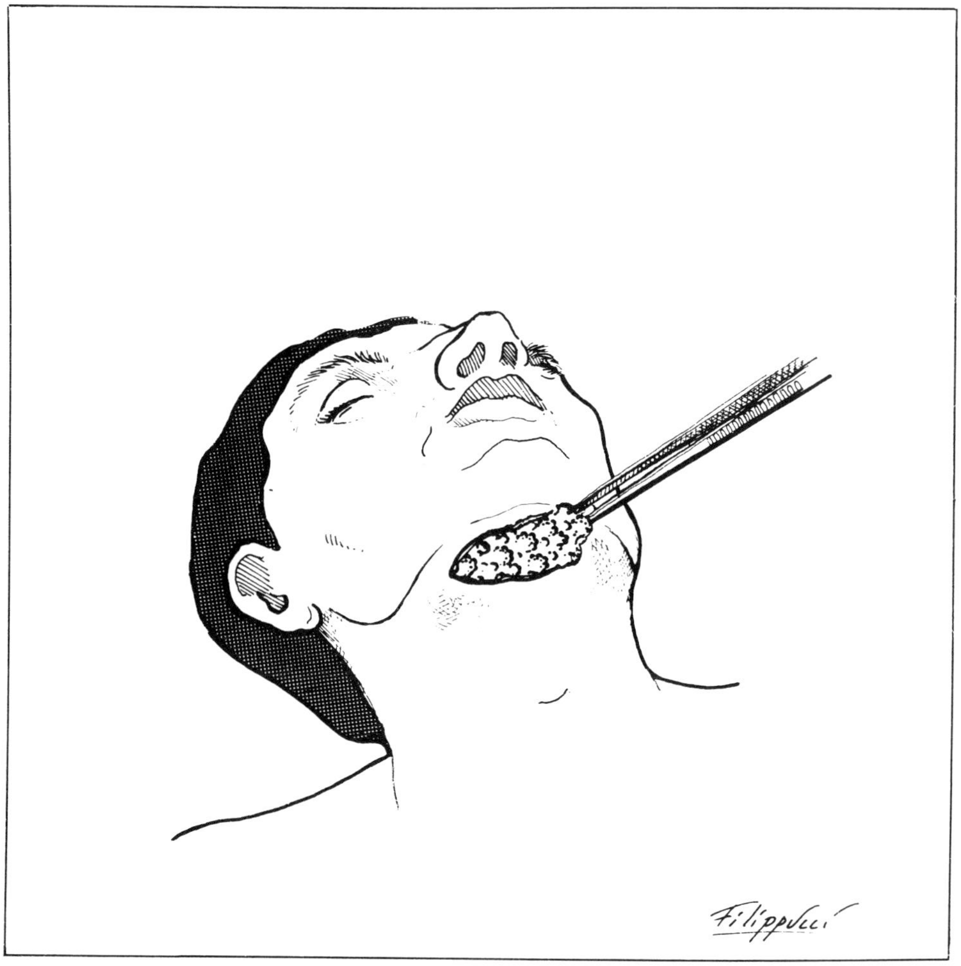

FIGURE 5: The redundant fat shown is removed from beneath the chin as a "chin tuck" *(submental lipectomy)* is performed.

CASE HISTORY

C.R. was a 32-year-old housewife who had been bothered by her pointy chin and a fullness beneath her chin which was present in spite of her very slender and athletic frame. She wished her double chin cleared and wanted something to be done to improve her pointed chin. She usually wore her hair down to cover her chin and neck.

Under local anesthesia in the office, the offending fat was tapered to give a clean neckline and a small chin implant was placed with more fullness at the sides than in the center. It was necessary to remove little skin. The patient was very satisfied with the result. Afterwards, she more frequently wore her hair up.

PREPARATION

The customary *Vitamin K and C are prescribed* and the patient advised to *avoid aspirin-containing products and Vitamin E for two weeks preoperatively*. The face is washed with *Phisohex*® on the morning of surgery and no make-up is worn. Men should shave on the morning of surgery. Per routine, *medical photographs are taken* to aid in the preoperative planning and help illustrate the possible need for chin augmentation.

The patient should set aside a week for the procedure; and unless extensive additional surgery is contemplated, most patients prefer local anesthesia and outpatient, office surgery for *submental lipectomy* or "chin tuck" with or without an *augmentation mentoplasty* or chin implant.

THE PROCEDURE

After preliminary sedation both by injection and intravenous, the chin area is numbed with local anesthesia. A short curvilinear incision is then made in the shadow-line beneath the chin.

The fat responsible for the double-chin or bulging neckline is removed with scissors and the margins of its removal delicately tapered into the surrounding fat to obtain a smooth, contoured result (see **Fig. 5**). Bleeding is controlled with cautery.

In many patients, the neck muscles *(platysma)* in this area may be widely separated as two separate bands (an anatomic variation) instead of being joined in the middle. To eliminate these bands, the front borders of the muscle may be sewn together.

If a chin implant is to be placed, a pocket is created over the chin to accommodate this implant which is placed directly over the bone. The implant is a solid silicon block sculpted and shaped as required for the patient's problem.

The skin of the neck is then drawn forward, so that any redundant skin from the neck will be brought to overlie the forward incision. This extra skin is removed and the incision closed in layers with individual stitches of fine suture material.

A bulky pressure dressing is placed, similar to that described for face-lifting; it is allowed to remain on overnight.

RECUPERATION

The bulky dressing is removed the following day. All sutures are removed by 7 days and the patient may be seen socially at this time. Any slight redness of the incision will fade over the next few weeks and may be easily covered by make-up.

PRECAUTIONS AND POTENTIAL COMPLICATIONS

Rarely, as in all facial surgery, bleeding may cause a *hematoma.* This blood may be evacuated in the office so that it does not mar the final result but will usually result in bruising that persists a few days longer.

If the surgeon is not skilful in tapering the margins of fat removal, irregularities or dimpling may result. This is best avoided by conservative and deliberate contouring of the fat excision.

FINISHING TOUCHES

That a further improvement in the profile might be gained by a small chin implant or *chin augmentation* was already mentioned. Improving the projection of the chin serves to help define the angle between the throat and chin.

Simultaneous surgery upon the *platysmal bands* was also mentioned as a way of removing neck bands at the time of *submental lipectomy*. Obviously, if there is cheek and neck sagging in addition to a fat pad or neck bands, *cheeklift* or *face and necklift* may be indicated as well to help define the jaw and neckline.

Cheek, face and necklifts have been discussed previously; *chin augmentation* and procedures upon the *platysma* or its overlying *fascia* will be discussed in future chapters.

* * *

CHAPTER 15

Altering Puffy Cheeks

Two related problems are discussed in this chapter. Although they have separate causes and require different treatments, they frequently occur together and are both amenable to outpatient, office surgery correction under local anesthesia.

The first problem tends to occur as a family trait and consists of a puffy-cheeked or round-faced appearance that is present without an accompanying generalized obesity. A substantial deposit of fat in the cheek itself causes the problem which is usually emphasized by cheek bones that are not very prominent. Treatment must be directed to the removal of redundant fat and recognizing when it is appropriate to further emphasize the cheek bones by augmentation.

The second problem tends to occur with aging and consists of very pronounced laughlines *(nasolabial folds)* that have developed into jowls in which there is a significant height difference between the cheek and the "muzzle" area of the face. This is emphasized by the receding changes that occur with age in the bones of the upper and lower jaw about the teeth. This height difference and jowl will only be partially alleviated by face or cheek lifting and may require local treatment for its eradication.

I almost never perform either of these procedures alone, nor do I perform cheek defatting for generalized obesity. Cautious cheek defatting is usually carried out to further improve cheek augmentation with or without cheeklift. Direct jowl surgery is carried out to remove what lifting procedures on the skin and muscle may have failed to correct. It is considered *only* in older patients with fair skins—those in whom incisions heal inconspicuously and may, if necessary, be subsequently dermabraded.

CASE HISTORY

L.N. was a 38-year-old singer who was just beginning to have some cheek sagging about her jawline. She had always had puffy cheeks and "invisible" cheek bones. She wished something to be done to improve her appearance which was very important in her line of work.

Under local anesthesia in the hospital (she had a "buttock tuck" performed during the same admission), a cheeklift *(meloplasty)* was performed, cheek implants inserted, and the cheek fat pads reduced.

The patient was so pleased with the results that she cut her hair in a pixie-ish style to go with her new look and had all her pictures retaken.

PREPARATION

Aspirin-containing products and Vitamin E should be avoided for two week preoperatively and *Vitamin C and Vitamin K are prescribed. Medical photographs* are particularly important in providing a means for preoperative discussion of patient's desires and surgeon's intents as well as their use in surgical planning and records.

Preoperative skin care should be meticulous along previously discussed lines, and the face is washed with *Phisohex®* on the morning of surgery.

THE PROCEDURE

Through the cheeklift incision described previously (along the front of the ear and behind the earlobe and ear), the cheek fat pad and the cheek bones are exposed and any lifting required can be performed.

If a puffy cheek is to be defatted, the fat pad is found in front of the strong muscle which closes the jaw *(masseter)* and fat may be gently teased out and removed. Great care must be taken not to injure the branches of the facial nerve to the mouth which are above the fat. I wear a special headlight for illumination when performing this procedure.

If a marked height difference and jowl remains after facelifting (which would include, in this case, a *SMAS* plication or resuspension to be discussed later), the offending area is excised in an elliptical pattern which is so planned that the resulting incision falls exactly into the laughline. This excision allows direct removal of any underlying cheek fat present. Care is taken not to injure any of the small branches of the facial nerve to the mouth in this area.

A bulky facelift dressing is placed and allowed to remain overnight. If a great deal of cheek-defatting has been performed, I place a suction drain which will also be removed the following morning.

RECUPERATION

The bulky dressing and drain, if any, are removed the following day. Laughline sutures are removed by the 5th postoperative day and any cheek-lift sutures are removed by 10 days postoperatively.

Generally two weeks are required for any bruising and swelling to subside. The face should be washed particularly gently afterwards for the first two weeks and sun should be avoided for 4–6 weeks unless a full sunblock with *PABA* is used.

PRECAUTIONS AND POTENTIAL COMPLICATIONS

As in all facial surgery, rarely, bleeding may cause a collection of blood or serum, termed a *hematoma* to occur. For this reason suction drains are employed. Evacuation of this blood usually requires a reopening of the incision in the case of cheek defatting.

Since fat occurs in a globular distribution, the surgeon must exercise deliberate care and be conservative in his excision or *asymmetry* may result. Correction would be achieved by further fat removal on the fuller side or silicon injection on the less full side.

If any of the fibers of the facial nerve are injured near the mouth during cheek defatting, several months will be required for a complete return of symmetry to the smile. Treatment is almost always conservative rather than surgical.

FINISHING TOUCHES

Possible *cheek bone augmentation* may be simultaneously performed to make the cheek bones appear higher or more pronounced. No additional time for convalescence is required and the result may be dramatically improved.

A *cheeklift* may clean up a jawline that has just begun to be obscured and so improve the facial balance. By redraping the skin more tautly, the cheeks tend to be less full beneath the cheek bones.

Occasionally, the midface may not be as far forward as aesthetically desireable although the bite is quite normal. Deep hollows are present in these patients beneath and at the sides of the nostrils. A small, U-shaped *maxillary implant* can be inserted at the base of the nose to lessen the height difference between cheek and "muzzle" in these cases to further improve the result.

When local jowl excisions have been used, *perioral dermabrasion*, generally carried out approximately 6 weeks postoperatively, will not only improve the laughline incisions, but will also remove the fine wrinkles about the mouth usually present in these patients.

* * *

PART II
FACEMAKING

B. Rearranging Facial Muscles

CHAPTER 16

Alleviating Eyelid Festoons and Crow's Feet

If you pinch your thumb against your forefinger, you will notice a few radiating wrinkles at the base of the thumb from the folding of extra skin. The crow's feet that accumulate at the corner of the eye originate for a somewhat similar reason as the surrounding circular muscle, the *orbicularis oculi*, closes the eye. With every smile, squint and blink, forces act to create wrinkles at the corners of the eyes. At first these crow's feet are present only during smiling; however, as time passes, they remain even in repose. As the forehead and eyebrows droop, extra skin is added, and these wrinkles become deeper and more pronounced.

During eyelid lift *(blepharoplasty)*, as described in previous chapters, the circular muscle at the corner of the eye can be treated in such a manner as to not only alleviate crow's feet, but also to reduce the forces causing them. This adds no time to that required for eyelid lift convalescence but does add to the immediate postoperative swelling.

In most older patients, it is desireable and flattering to suspend a slip of muscle from the lower eyelid a little higher on the bone to give a slight lift to the corner of the eye and so create an "almond eye". This makes up for the laxity that develops in the lower lid with age that tends to create a "rounder" eye.

In many young patients, particularly among those who habitually squint and in some of those who wear contacts, the muscle surrounding the eye develops so well that there is an unattractive horizontal bulge of muscle termed a *festoon*. It can be differentiated from fatty bags by its firmness and

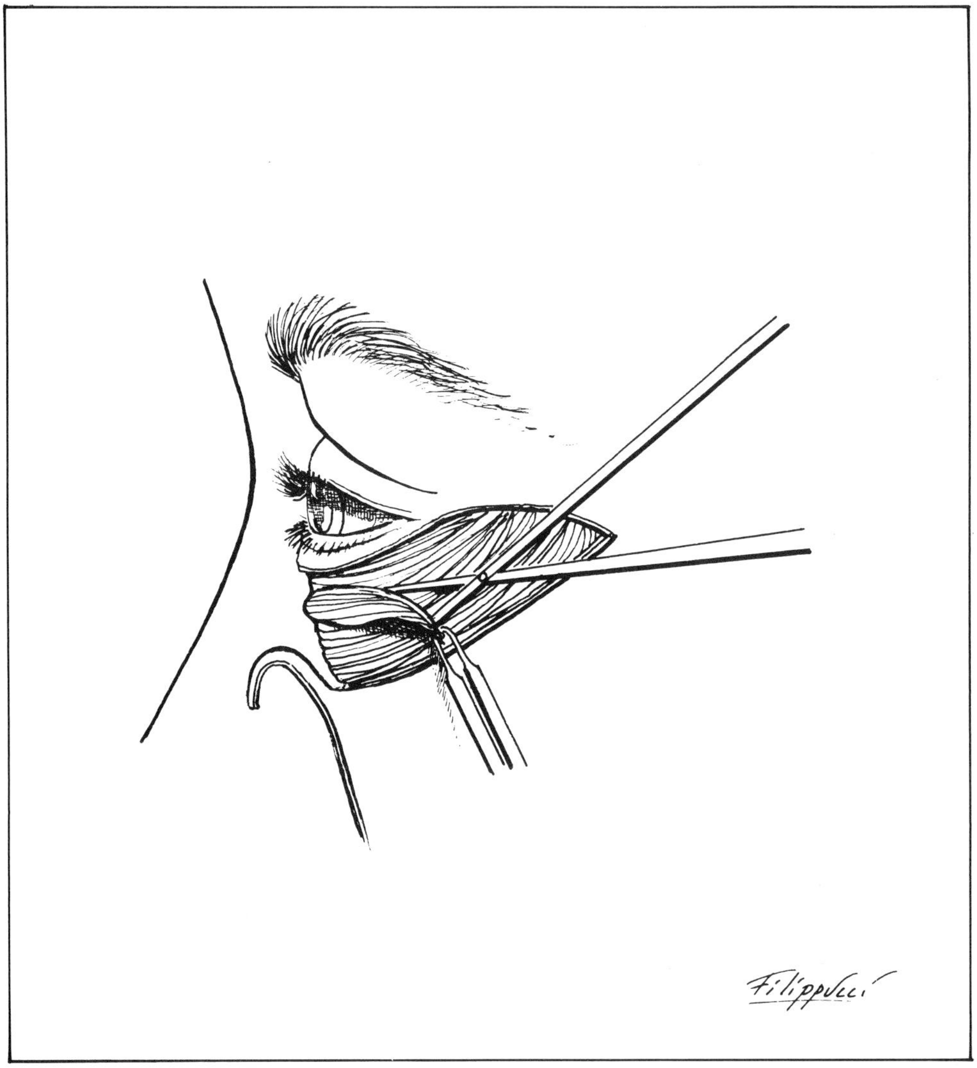

FIGURE 6: Overly-developed eyelid muscle responsible for an eyelid festoon is removed to sculpt a flat eyelid.

the fact that it is more pronounced with smiling. If a strip of this muscle is removed at the time of eyelid lift, this festoon can be eliminated.

Other procedures upon the eye muscles, when indicated, would include lifting a droopy lid by shortening the muscle which lifts the upper lid *(levator palpebrae superioris)* and "Westernizing" the Oriental eye. An Occidental upper eyelid fold *(supratarsal fold)* can be created by a *supratarsal fixation* in which the muscle is attached to the skin as it is normally in Western or "double" eyes.

These modifications of eyelid lift to include procedures upon the underlying muscle have originated in recent years to improve and enhance the results of traditional skin and fat-only eyelid surgery. They do not add much operating time to the procedure, still allow local anesthesia and outpatient surgery, and do not require additional time for convalescence.

CASE HISTORY

K.D. was a bubbly 42-year-old housewife who was disturbed by multiple crow's feet and lower eyelid bags. It bothered her to smile, because she felt the crow's feet gave away her age. On examination, she also had muscle festoons, some fatty out-pocketing, and redundant skin *(blepharochalasis)*.

Under local anesthesia in the office, redundant skin and fat were removed, the strip of muscle causing the festoon excised, and the muscle causing the crow's feet mostly divided and repositioned. The patient was very pleased with the result and then felt she could again smile freely without being self-conscious.

PREPARATION

As for all eyelid surgery, *aspirin-containing products and Vitamin E are avoided for two weeks preoperatively*, and *Vitamin K and Vitamin C are prescribed. Medical photographs* are integral to the preoperative evaluation and planning. The face is washed with *Phisohex*.® and no make-up, contact lens, or false eyelashes are worn on the day of surgery.

THE PROCEDURE

If there is a lower eyelid festoon present, the strip of muscle causing it is lifted with forceps and excised with scissors (see **Fig. 6**). Any bleeding is

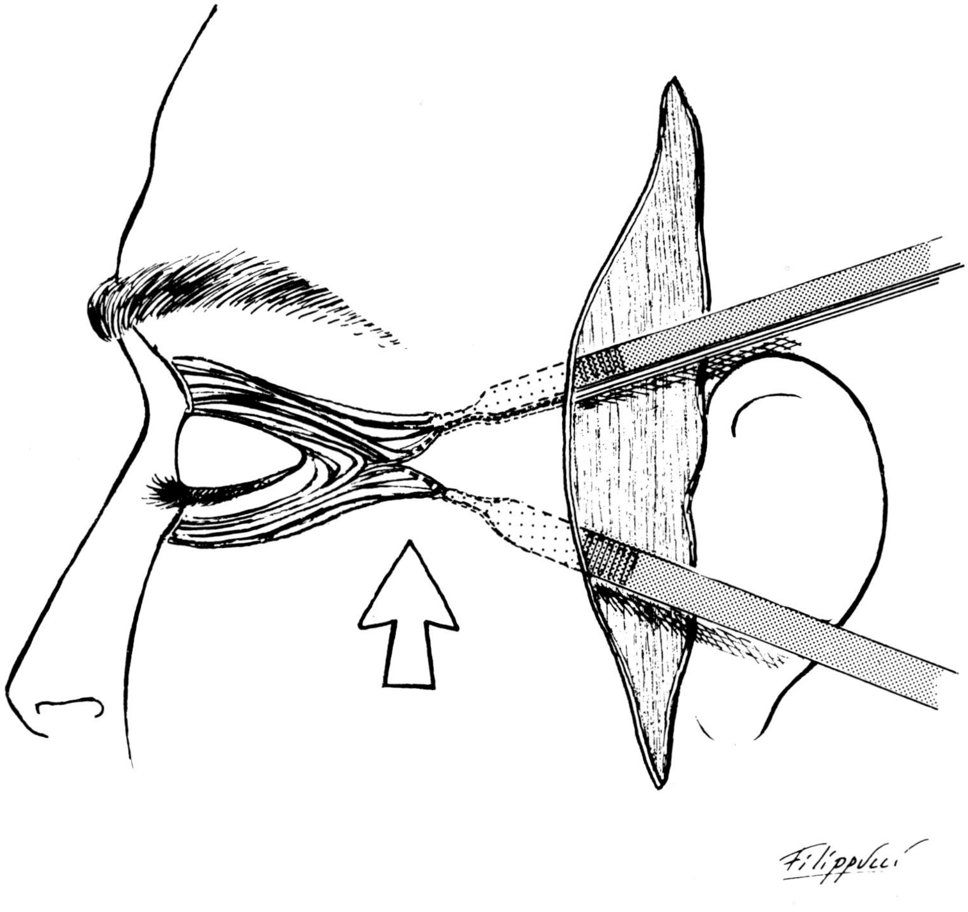

FIGURE 7: The arrow points to the partial division and spreading out of the eyelid muscle at the corner of the eye to eliminate crow's feet. Access is shown through the incision for a facelift which is being performed concurrently.

controlled with needle-point cautery. On many occasions, I will raise the lower eyelid flap *deep* to this offending portion of muscle rather than just beneath the skin, so that this festoon is automatically included with resected skin. This approach has the advantage that less bruising is visible through the skin since dissection is at a deeper level.

At the outer corner of the eye, the circular muscle surrounding it *(orbicularis oculi)* is partially divided in a horizontal direction, beginning at its most peripheral fibers. It is flattened, spread out, and held in this position by several stitches of fine absorbable suture. Somewhat greater tension and slight upward lift may be placed upon the lower portion of muscle if this is desired. **Fig. 7** depicts this procedure being carried out through a facelift incision since it is commonly performed concurrently on these patients.

The incisions are closed as described for eyelid lift, and iced compresses are immediately applied to the eyelids.

RECUPERATION

Iced compresses for the first few days are helpful in preventing bruising and swelling. All sutures are removed by the third day and make-up may be worn four days after suture removal, providing it is *completely removed at night with a gentle cleanser.* As for most eyelid surgery, generally two weeks should be set aside before tinted glasses can be discarded socially.

Direct sunlight should be avoided for four weeks unless darkly tinted or mirrored sunglasses are worn. Sunburn causes the freshly operated eyelid to swell.

PRECAUTIONS AND POTENTIAL COMPLICATIONS

The potential complications are the same as for eyelid lifts, namely, *milia*, *hematoma*, and *ectropion*. The treatments are also the same. The whitehead-like inclusion cysts that may occur along the suture line are termed *milia* and may be easily removed during postoperative visits. Bleeding may occur rarely and cause an accumulation of blood or *hematoma*; this may be evacuated and usually only results in a temporary increase in bruising. *Ectropion*, a slight turning or pulling away of the lower lid from the eye, usually responds to a supporting steristrip for a week or two. However, this is even more uncommon than in routine eyelifts if the muscle supporting the lower lid was resuspended as the "muscle sling" described above.

FINISHING TOUCHES

Since the cartilage which supports the lower lid weakens with time and gives a more round eye with age, suspending the muscle of the lower lid at a slightly higher level has the advantage of restoring a more youthful or "almond" eye shape. In older patients, the cartilage may have become very thinned. A part of it may be removed as a "tarsal tuck" *(Kuhnt-Szymanowski procedure)* to tone up a lax lower lid.

Removal of any skin or fat redundancy is routinely carried out concurrently. Treating any associated eyebrow sag with a *forehead lift* will further enhance any surgical treatment of upper eyelid redundancy and crow's feet.

If the face is flat, *cheek implants* can be placed to help alleviate the deep furrows beneath eyelid bags as well as improve facial aesthetics. The results of these combined procedures can be far more dramatic than the individual procedures carried out separately.

* * *

CHAPTER 17

Improving Jowls and Turkey Gobblers

When the laughlines *(nasolabial folds)* deepen with age and begin to cover the jawline, jowls are formed. As skin becomes redundant beneath the chin on the throat, very unattractive folds may be formed which hang down and may resemble "turkey gobblers". Both jowls and turkey gobblers are only partly removed by a traditional "skin-only" facelift. To eliminate these severe signs of aging, procedures must be performed upon the facial musculature beneath.

The corresponding muscle to that which shakes off fleas in horses exists only on the face and neck of humans and is called the *platysma*. There is a relatively strong overlying fibrous layer which is called the Superficial Musculo-Aponeurotic System, or *SMAS* for short. To eliminate a marked jowl, sutures may be placed in the SMAS to imbricate and tighten it *(SMAS plication)*; thereby less tension is placed upon the skin. In more severe cases, the *platysma* may be partially or even totally divided and resuspended to give a cleaner jawline and neck *("platysma lift")*. If the platysma of the two sides of the neck is separated in the middle, an anatomic variation that may result in neck bands, it may be sewn together so that a sling is created to retain a youthful neck. Buttressing the muscle support beneath the chin greatly improves facelifting results in this area.

It may occasionally be necessary to directly remove portions of neck skin at the site of the offending turkey gobblers with incisions placed in the neck crease in addition to or instead of the more routine beneath-the-chin incision for *submental lipectomy* or "chin tuck". Fortunately, *SMAS plication* or *platysma lift* usually can avoid this.

For a limited *SMAS plication*, I will still perform facelift in the office; however, for a formal *platysma lift*, I prefer the hospital. If a great deal of work is to be required to clean up the neckline, I usually prefer general anesthesia instead of local.

Both procedures add significantly to the immediate postoperative swelling. They usually do not increase the amount of bruising; in fact, since the dissection for *platysma lift* occurs at a deeper level, bruising is usually less. The usual period of time to allot for convalescence from this modified facelift remains at about 2 weeks.

CASE HISTORY

B.R. was a 72-year-old house wife who had marked jowls, a severely crepey neck, upper and lower eyelid bags, multiple fine wrinkles about the mouth and cheeks. She was slender and healthy but felt her looks classified her as an old lady even though she walked about 10 blocks every day.

Under local anesthesia in the hospital, her upper and lower lids were lifted, a facelift with a *SMAS plication*, and a *submental lipectomy* were performed. Four weeks later, her entire face was chemically peeled.

The postoperative improvement was dramatic. Although she appeared "spunky" before surgery, the patient seemed even more energetic afterwards. She was most pleased that she was no longer "type cast" by her looks into the Nursing Home or Retirement Community age-group. She still preferred golf to bridge! She was reminded to wear a sunblock on the golf course.

PREPARATION

As usual, *aspirin-containing products and Vitamin E are avoided for two weeks before surgery* and *Vitamin K and Vitamin C are prescribed. Medical photographs* facilitate preoperative planning. Chin-up views with clenched teeth are particularly illustrative of neck bands. *Phisohex®* is used for facewash and shampoo before surgery.

I will have a detailed discussion with any patients upon whom I believe supplementary direct-approach neck incisions might be necessary. In some cases I may merely prepare the patient so that we can decide together later if it might be worth a neck crease incision for additional improvement of a bad turkey gobbler deformity.

THE PROCEDURE

Before surgery, I will have the patient clench his or her teeth with the chin lifted to illustrate the front borders of *platysma* and any neck bands requiring direct attention. I will mark the location of these on the skin as well as any fat deposits requiring contouring.

If a *SMAS plication* is to be performed, after the facelift incisions and sufficient skin underming have been performed, lines of sutures of absorbable material are placed beneath the cheek bones and in front of and beneath the ear to flatten out the jowl. Suction drains are placed and the incisions closed as described for facelift.

If a *platysma lift* is to be performed, skin underming is more limited, this muscle is incised and undermined in front of and below the ear (see **Fig. 8**). Great care is taken to visualize and preserve all branches of the facial nerve which come up through the parotid salivary gland and branch into the *platysma* from is under-surface. When required to give a crisp neckline, the muscle is transected completely about one half of the way down the neck (at the level of the next cartilage below the "Adam's apple"). If it is split or redundant in the middle, it is sewn together and imbricated if necessary to make a taut, contiguous sling. The muscle is then lifted up and back and sewn into its new position with interrupted sutures. Suction drains are placed and the facelift incisions closed routinely.

RECUPERATION

Convalescence from these procedures is similar to that for facelift except the immediate postoperative swelling is usually more pronounced. Bruising is usually less in the *platysma lifts* since the dissection is at a deeper level.

Most patients say they are aware of a tightness on turning their neck from side to side which persists several weeks. This rarely causes any significant postoperative discomfort.

Direct sunlight should be avoided for 4 weeks unless a full sunblock is used since it will exacerbate and prolong swelling. The face should be washed gently in an upwards direction.

Temporarily numb earlobes and areas of the scalp warrant being careful of wearing time for heavy earrings and using low settings on hair driers and blowers to avoid unfelt injury until normal sensation returns.

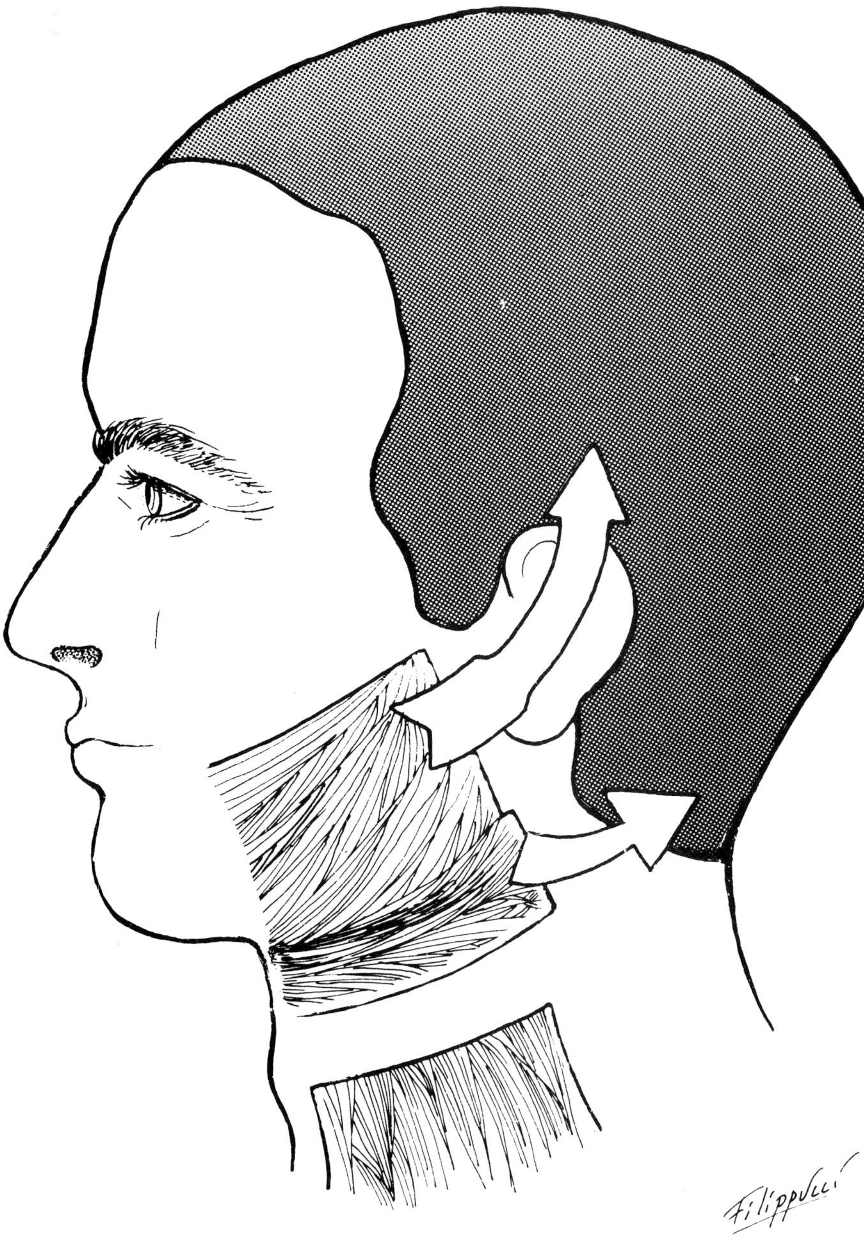

FIGURE 8: The *platysma* is sectioned in the neck and its fibers re-directed (as shown by the arrows) to give a sharp neck and jawline as a *platysma lift* is performed.

PRECAUTIONS AND POTENTIAL PROBLEMS

The potential problems discussed previously in facelifting, namely *hematoma, infection*, and *scarring* still rarely occur with these modified procedures and are treated in the same manner. Bad scarring occurs even less frequently since there is less tension placed upon the skin.

Nerve injury is a somewhat greater consideration because of the proximity of dissection to the branches of the facial nerve. However, its occurrence has not been significantly greater with these modified facelifts. Treatment, in most cases, would still be non-operative, awaiting spontaneous return of function.

Minor contour irregularities may result from the muscle surgery on the neck. They usually resolve with time. The surgeon must exercise caution when operating on thick-necked individuals to avoid "skeletonizing" the neck and to avoid "masculinizing" a woman's neck by making the "Adam's apple" more prominent. For this reason, I generally will not perform a *platysma lift* on a bull-necked individual. In women, if I do completely sever the *platysma*, I will do it at the level of the *cricoid cartilage*—the next one beneath the *thyroid cartilage* which has the "Adam's apple"—so as not to make the "Adam's apple" more prominent.

FINISHING TOUCHES

Eyelid lift is routinely carried out at the time of face and necklift because the aging changes about the eyes become even more apparent by contrast with a youthfulized face and neck.

The advantage of *chin augmentation* in further improving the necklines of some patients has been previously mentioned as have *perioral peels* and *dermabrasions* for removing fine wrinkles about the mouth. Also mentioned previously were correction of the subtle signs of aging—*lifting droopy nasal tips* and *reducing large earlobes*.

* * *

CHAPTER 18

Softening Frowns and Scowls

Foreheads are most expressive. When we concentrate, our forehead muscles tense; indeed, this is one of the frequent causes of headaches. When our faces communicate surprise, approval or disapproval, our foreheads do much of this silent speaking.

At first these forehead wrinkles and scowl lines between the eyes are present only when we call upon the underlying muscles for expression. However, in time they do not completely disappear in repose. When vertical scowl lines between the eyebrows add a fixed, stern look to the face, the face communicates an emotion that may not be present. Many young men and women seek correction of this condition.

Forehead wrinkles begin to take up residence when we enter our late 20's and constitute one of the earliest signs of aging. As with scowl lines, they first are present *only* during facial animation. However, they soon disappear incompletely when the face is at rest. They can become a fixed frown and suggest an unhappy background or past. What is worse, they can remind one of whatever caused them in the first place! If they are present only because of an unusual pattern of facial expression, they are even more undesireable because they communicate false messages. For these reasons, many patients consult the plastic surgeon.

In an earlier chapter, we discussed forehead lifts for sagging eyebrows, horizontal wrinkles at the root of the nose, and to help alleviate crow's feet.

To eliminate frown and scowl lines, we have two available remedies. The first is appropriate for earlier lines which are just beginning to become permanent; this is *collagen injection.* If the pattern of facial expression is altered, this non-operative mode may be sufficient.

The areas of dermal and subcutaneous thinning at the sites of the wrinkles are "beefed up" with injections of collagen *(Zyderm®).* As with all collagen treatments, a skin test is done first to rule out the possibility of allergy. In most early cases, one or two treatments are sufficient. Early forehead wrinkles and scowl lines can be eliminated by this means. However, it is impractical to use this method for more advanced cases because of the multitude of injections, amount of collagen, and number of treatments that would be required. It should also be emphasized, that *unless the habit of facial expression is changed, these wrinkles will recur.* Just as if you were to place a piece of cardboard behind a pleat in a curtain, the curtain will eventually crease right next to the cardboard buttress if you keep it folded to the side of a window.

In more advanced cases, and when the patient cannot change his or her pattern of expression, a *forehead lift* with excision of a strip of the underlying muscle *(frontalis)* and sectioning of the muscles responsible for scowl lines *(corrugators)* is required. This can usually be performed in the office under local anesthesia. If I am concurrently treating significant eyebrow sag and desire to even obtain a little lift to a droopy nasal tip in an older patient, the more extensive undermining required leads me to prefer general anesthesia with an overnight hospitalization.

CASE HISTORY

M.J. was an attractive 39-year-old woman who had been down on Wall Street since her early 20's. The tension of her job had taken its toll. Deep vertical scowl lines and three or four marked forehead wrinkles marred her youthful face which was graced with creamy, well-cared-for skin. There was just the start of an upper eyelid skin redundancy which only showed when she was tired. The patient sought correction of her forehead wrinkles and scowl lines.

Under local anesthesia in the office, a forehead lift was performed which eliminated the slight redundancy of upper lid skin, a strip of forehead muscle was removed to eliminate the frown lines, and the offending muscles were sectioned to eliminate the scowl lines.

The patient was very pleased with her "softened" and "more relaxed" appearance. She felt her forehead no longer gave away the history of her trading stresses. In addition, the rejuvenating effect upon her upper eyelids made her look more rested.

PREPARATION

In men undergoing this procedure, I will always attempt to ascertain the likelihood for balding by inquiry into their family history. I can protect against a mild temporal recession by curving the incision quite far back in the hairline. However, if more than average temple balding is likely I discourage the procedure unless the patient desires to keep up with any future recession with hair transplants.

Women should bleach or tint their hair a few days before surgery because a touch-up is not allowed until 3 weeks after surgery. The hair is shampooed with *Phisohex*® the night before surgery. No hair spray or grooming aid is worn on the morning of surgery.

As per routine, *Vitamin C and Vitamin K are prescribed* and *Vitamin E and aspirin-containing products are to be avoided for two weeks preoperatively. Medical photographs* aid in preoperative planning and accurate records.

THE PROCEDURE

After injection of local anesthesia, a curved incision is made approximately 3 inches behind the hairline (see **Fig. 3**). The scalp and underlying muscle are then elevated and lifted to the degree required for correction of any associated eyebrow sag. Bleeding is controlled with cautery.

One or several strips of forehead muscle *(frontalis)* are removed as dictated by the severity of the problem. The short muscles causing scowl lines *(corrugators)* are divided and a portion of them removed to prevent their function.

The scalp is then reapproximated, removing any redundancy as required, and sewn with individual sutures in two layers. The underlying tissue is sewn with sutures that dissolve with time and the skin is closed with blue plastic sutures that are easy to see for removal. I do not like the staples some plastic surgeons use because they make it difficult for the patient to wash, comb or brush his or her hair.

A bulky dressing is placed after the procedure is finished and allowed to remain on until the following morning.

RECUPERATION

The dressing is removed on the following morning. In four or five days the patient may shampoo his or her hair (again with *Phisohex*®) and gently towel dry and brush it.

There is usually considerable swelling and some bruising about the eyelids which takes between one to two weeks to disappear. For this reason, the patient should set aside two weeks for the procedure.

All stitches are removed at 10 days. The patient may groom his or her hair normally at this time but should avoid bleaching, tinting or a permanent wave for an additional 7 to 10 days. Since portions of the scalp may be temporarily numb, low settings should be used on hair driers or blowers to prevent unfelt burns to the scalp.

PRECAUTIONS AND POTENTIAL PROBLEMS

Broadening of the scar should not occur if the underlying tissue was well-sewn. However, if it does, the scar may be revised in the office under local anesthesia.

A collection of blood (a *hematoma*) may occur rarely as it can in all surgery. Such a collection most frequently occurs within the first 24 hours and may be evacuated usually only with removal of a few sutures.

Since hair is difficult to sterilize, an *infection* may occur rarely and would be managed with appropriate antibiotics locally, by mouth, and if necessary by vein.

FINISHING TOUCHES

Any eyebrow sag is corrected concurrently. A droopy nasal tip in an older patient may be lifted at the same time. If the upper lids are being improved by the forehead lift, it may be appropriate to perform a *lower eyelid lift* to remove any lower eyelid bags.

A not infrequent combination of procedures is a cheeklift *(meloplasty)*, a forehead lift and lower eyelid lift. All three areas of the face are thus corrected in a younger individual not requiring much improvement upon the neck.

If early wrinkles are being treated non-surgically with collagen, it may be appropriate to lessen smile lines *(nasolabial folds)* with collagen at the same time. Beginning cheek hollows beneath the lower lids *(nasojugal folds)* may be also softened with collagen injections until corrective surgery is actually required.

In older, light-skinned patients, a *chemical peel* may be appropriate to remove the finer criss-crossing wrinkles that are not affected by forehead lift. Collagen injections can also be employed for this purpose in more olive-skinned patients.

* * *

PART II
FACEMAKING

C. Solid Tissue Sculpting

CHAPTER 19

Enlarging the Eye

Not infrequently, a patient will present with a prominent rim on the top, outer portion of the eye socket which makes the eye look smaller and slightly downcast. This is usually a family trait and has nothing at all to do with age. Removing a portion of this over-hanging bone has a remarkable opening and "cheering up" effect upon the eye.

Through the eyelid incision described for *blepharoplasty*, the bony rim is exposed and gently reduced with a fine rotating diamond burr. A fraction of an inch in this area counts a lot. Any offending fat or redundant skin is removed at the same time. Sutures are removed by the third or fourth day. Local anesthesia in the office provides suitable comfort and safety. Bruising is usually somewhat greater than for routine eyelid lift but generally resolves within the same two week period required for convalescence.

It is not uncommon to have an associated eyebrow sag compound the effect of a "shrinking eye" in an older patient. Concurrent forehead lift can greatly enhance the result in these patients. Any lower eyelid bags and crow's feet would usually be removed at the same time by appropriate surgery.

CASE HISTORY

R.S. was a 38-year-old translator. Her eyes had always had a melancholy appearance which had become worse as redundant skin had caused some hooding above her upper lashes. She had difficulty applying makeup to the outer portions of her eyelids and wanted something done to improve her appearance.

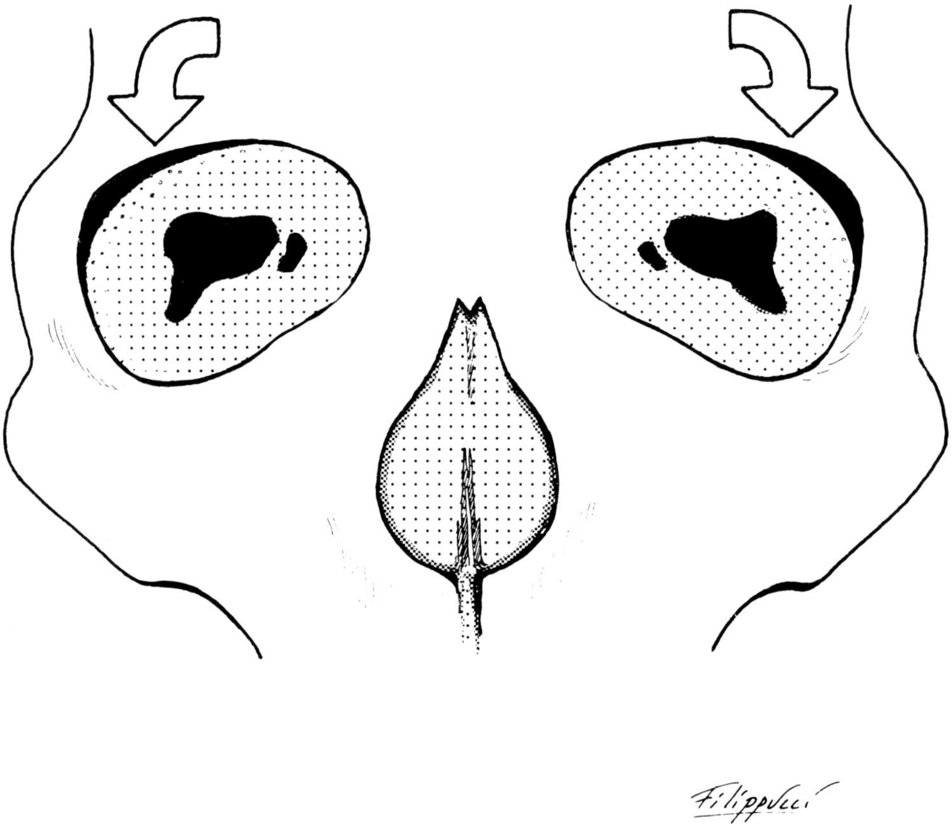

FIGURE 9: The arrows point to the overhanging portion of orbital rim that may be safely removed to "open up" the eye.

Under local anesthesia in the office, redundant upper lid skin and fat were removed. A portion of the bone at the upper, outer rim of the eye socket was removed to eliminate the down-sloping appearance.

The patient was very much pleased with the result and found it much easier to apply make-up in the mornings. She discarded her glasses for contact lens and felt she had a much "brighter" and "happier" look about her eyes.

PREPARATION

As customary, *Vitamin E and aspirin-containing products are avoided for two weeks preoperatively*, and *Vitamin K and Vitamin C are prescribed. Medical photographs* aid in preoperative planning.

The face is washed with *Phisohex*® on the morning of surgery and no make-up, contact lens or false eyelashes are worn.

THE PROCEDURE

After preliminary sedation and intravenous relaxants, local anesthetic is injected and redundant skin removed from the upper lid. The skin and muscle about the upper lid is retracted to expose the bony rim (see **Fig. 9**).

The overlying membrane *(periosteum)* is incised for about an inch and gently raised. A fine rotating burr, similar to a dentist's drill, is used to remove about 1/16 to 1/4″ of bone at the outer, upper portion of the eye socket rim.

The *periosteum* is reapproximated with fine individual stitches of absorbable suture and the eyelid skin closed as for eyelid lift. Iced compresses are immediately applied.

RECUPERATION

Iced compresses are continued for the next two days and all sutures are removed by the fourth day. Hypoallergenic make-up can be worn 4 days later provided it is carefully and completely removed at night with a gentle cleanser.

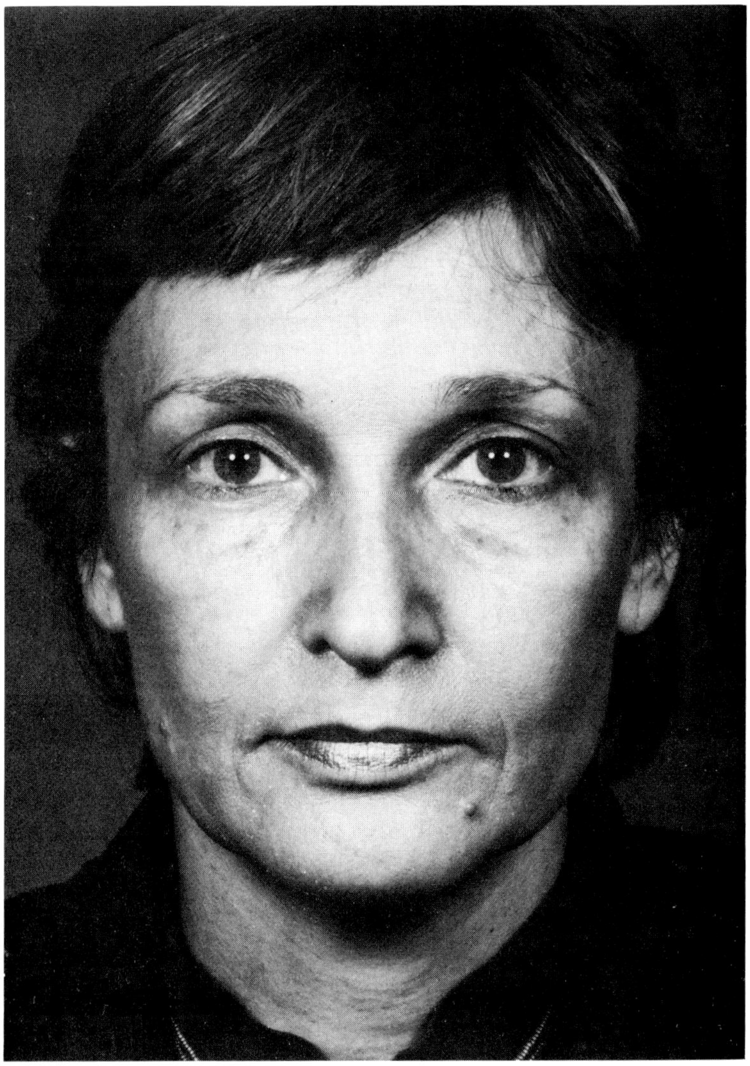

PHOTO 7: A patient with redundant upper and lower eyelid skin, deep *nasojugal folds* and a broad nasal bridge.

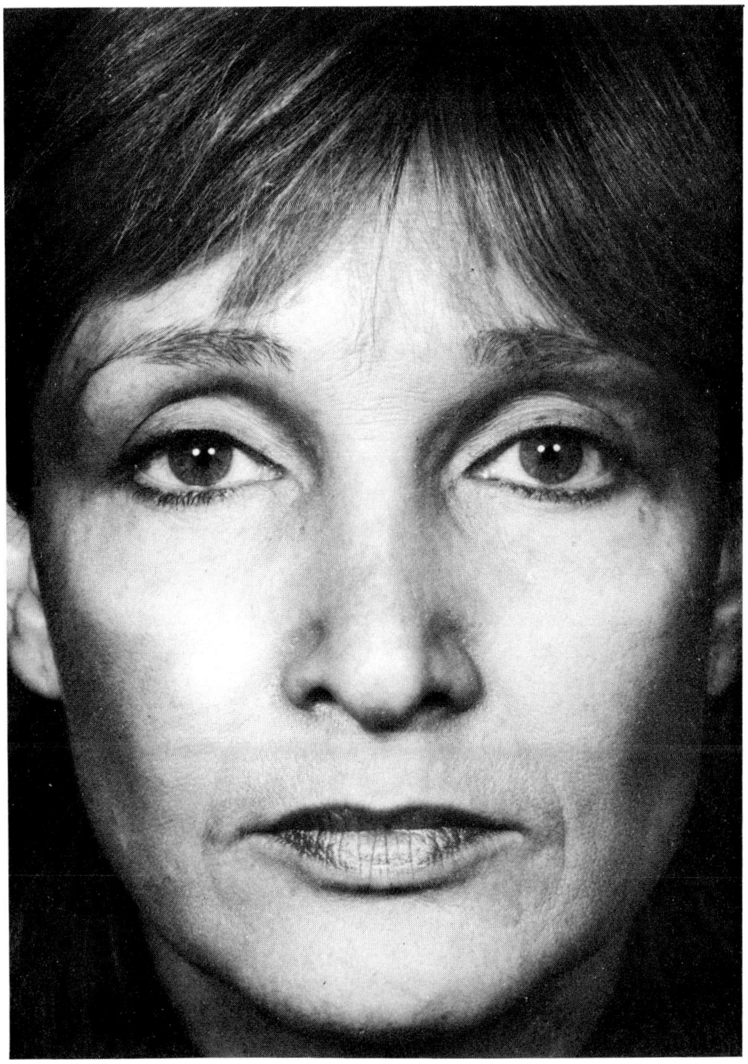

PHOTO 8: The same patient after *blepharoplasty* and *rhinoplasty* (and excision of mole on her left chin).

Bruising is almost always completely resolved by the end of the second week. The sun should be avoided for 4 weeks afterwards unless dark or mirrored sunglasses are worn.

PRECAUTIONS AND POTENTIAL COMPLICATIONS

Milia (whitehead-like cysts along the incision), *hematoma* (an accumulation of blood) and *scarring* are potential complications, which occur rarely as they do in all eyelid surgery and are treated as discussed previously. They occur no more frequently with "bony expansion" than they do with routine *blepharoplasty* (eyelid lift).

FINISHING TOUCHES

Removing any redundant fat, skin and muscle in both upper and lower lids is routinely carried out. Marked crow's feet are dealt with concurrently as are marked hollows beneath lower eyelid bags *(nasojugal folds)*.

Alluded to previously was the utilization of a *forehead lift* to treat any coexistant eyebrow sag. When appropriate, lifting the eyebrow and bony expansion work together to open and enhance the eyes.

If the nasal bridge is broader than ideal for the face, the eyes will have greater impact and appear larger if the nasal bridge is rendered more appropriate for the face with *rhinoplasty*. The broad "divider" detracts from the eyes as does a nasal hump (see **Photos 7** and **8**).

* * *

CHAPTER 20

Treating Receded Chins and Flat Faces

To give the most flattering profile, the chin should be close to a vertical line dropped from the angle between the root of the nose and the forehead. If the chin is much behind the line, it gives the appearance of being "weak" or receded and lends to premature jowling. This situation is easily remedied by an *augmentation mentoplasty* in which a solid silicon implant is sculpted to add prominence to the chin.

In some patients, the problem is greater than just a receded chin and consists of the lower jaw being too small or too far back so that the bite is poor. In these patients it may be necessary to section the jaw and slide the front fragment forward to restore a normal bite *(mandibular advancement)*. This is a more involved procedure and requires careful planning, Xrays, dental models, general anesthesia, hospitalization, and the combined efforts of a plastic surgeon and orthodontist. Afterwards, the teeth must be wired together for 6 weeks. Fortunately, most patients with receded chins do not have abnormal bites so that simple silicon implants suffice to correct the problem.

When chin augmentation is performed as a solitary procedure, I will place the implant through the mouth so that no outside incisions need be used. The internal sutures dissolve and need not be removed. Elastic tapes are placed on the skin to assure approximation of the implant to the bone and the overlying skin; these are crucial to the final result and allowed to remain in position for 5–7 days.

The patient will brush his or her lower teeth gently and take a fluid diet on the evening of surgery. The following day a soft diet, requiring little chewing, is recommended. There is usually very little bruising but generally the swelling takes about a week to resolve. The patient may be seen socially at this time although the lower lip may still be a little "stiff". Broad spectrum antibiotics are prescribed for a week postoperatively since the mouth contains many bacteria.

If a "chin tuck" or *submental lipectomy* is being performed concurrently, I will use the beneath-the-chin incision for placement of the implant to avoid a second incision.

A second, even more unattractive deformity, and I use that term because we are closer to reconstructive surgery than aesthetic plastic surgery when we correct it, is that of the flat face or "dish-face" appearance. This patient may have a totally normal bite (upper and lower teeth meet correctly) but does not have as much projection to the center portion of the face as normal. The lower lip seems very much more prominent than the flat upper lip, the tip of the nose is usually not very projecting, and there usually are deep hollows on either side of the nostrils. The overall effect is not very flattering.

Mid-face flatness or "dish-face" deformity can be corrected by a "U-shaped" implant inserted about the base of the nose to add prominence and projection to the mid-face. The tip and base of the nose may be lifted, the upper lip brought forward, and the hollows beneath and to the sides of the nostrils lessened. If only *maxillary augmentation* is being performed, I carve this solid silicon implant to achieve the desired effect at the time of surgery and insert it through the mouth. If nasal surgery is being performed concurrently, as it frequently is, I insert it through one of the intranasal incisions instead.

The procedure usually requires between 6 and 8 days of convalescence for the swelling to subside. I usually employ local anesthesia and office surgery unless medical problems dictate otherwise. As with chin augmentation, the sutures dissolve and need not be removed.

In severe cases of "dish-face" deformity, the upper teeth will be abnormally far back and the bite will be off. In these cases the bones of the mid-face need be surgically advanced to correct the problem. As with mandibular advancement, this is a much more involved procedure requiring general anesthesia, hospitalization, Xrays, dental models, and the combined efforts of the plastic surgeon and orthodontist. The teeth need to be wired together for 6 weeks. This is called *mid-face* or *maxillary advancement* and is never performed solely for reasons of cosmesis but for orthodontic reasons as well. For most patients, simple implants suffice to adequately correct the problem.

After mid-face augmentation, a fluid diet is suggested for the first post-operative day and a soft diet for the following day so that chewing can be avoided. I always prescribe broad-spectrum antibiotics since it is difficult to "sterilize" the mouth.

CASE HISTORY

M.A. was a 22-year-old ballet dancer who principally wanted something done to improve her profile. She had a very receded chin and a nasal hump. On the front view, the nose was somewhat broad but this did not detract markedly from her appearance. She felt her profile hurt her when she was on stage.

Under local anesthesia in the office, *rhinoplasty* and *augmentation mentoplasty* were performed. The nasal hump was removed and the nose narrowed. The chin was brought forward with a shaped silicon implant placed through the mouth.

The patient was very pleased with her improved profile and liked her front view much better as well. She found added confidence during her subsequent dancing. The first thing she did after surgery was to have her company pictures retaken.

PREPARATION

The usual *Vitamin K and C are prescribed* while *Vitamin E and aspirin-containing products are avoided for 2 weeks preoperatively. Medical Photographs* are essential for preoperative planning. *Xrays* may occasionally be required to elucidate unusual conditions and are always required for *mandibular* or *mid-face advancement. Dental models* are also required in either of these latter two procedures.

The face is washed with *Phisohex®*, the teeth are brushed, and the mouth rinsed with hydrogen peroxide and Listerine® on the morning of surgery. No make-up, contacts or false eyelashes are worn. If the patient wears dentures, these should be worn to the office. Several types very much influence the lips.

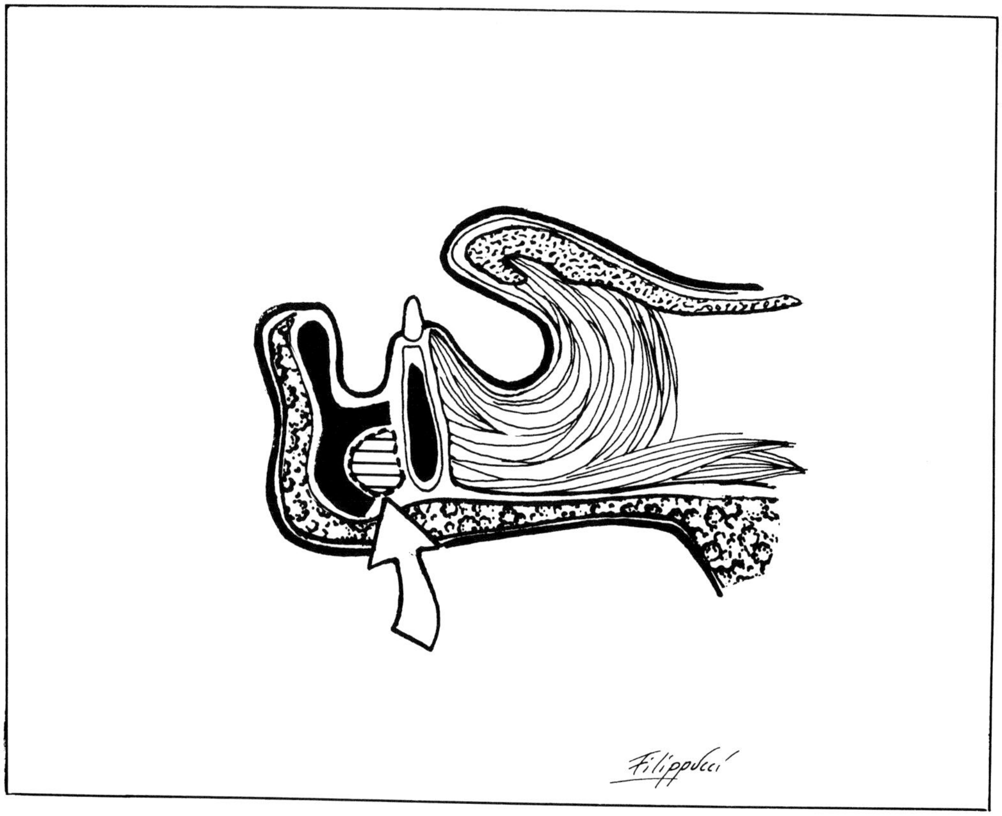

FIGURE 10: The arrow shows the proper placement of the implant in front of the jaw to make a receded chin more prominent *(augmentation mentoplasty).*

THE PROCEDURE

Chin augmentation: After numbing the area in front of the lower incisors with local anesthetic, a small incision is made in the crease between gum and lip. Blunt spreading between the two muscles which evert the lower lip allows access to the chin. A pocket is created for the implant above the bone (see **Fig. 10**). The implant is carved to achieve the desired effect and lodge on the slight bony prominence in the midline. Any bleeding is controlled with electrocautery.

The muscles and *mucosa* (lining of the mouth) are closed with individual sutures that dissolve in 2–3 weeks. Elastic tapes are placed upon the skin to assure that the implant remains closely approximated to the bone and overlying skin.

Mid-face augmentation: After numbing the area with local anaesthetic, a small incision is made above the upper incisors slightly to the left of midline. (I am right-handed.) The area about the base of the nostrils is bluntly freed. A slightly U-shaped solid silicon implant is carved to size and inserted (see **Fig. 11**). It is so carved that it lodges in place and is anchored on a bony prominence called the *nasal spine*.

Bleeding is minimal, but that which occurs is controlled with cautery. The mucosal "keyhole" is sewn with individual sutures that dissolve.

RECUPERATION

For either chin or mid-face augmentation, the patient will take a fluid diet for the evening of surgery. The following day a soft diet is permitted. The front teeth should be brushed gently and the mouth rinsed with a mix of salt water and hydrogen peroxide after meals and at bedtime for the first 3 days. A broad-spectrum antibiotic, generally *Keflex®*, is prescribed since the mouth cannot be rendered totally free of germs. In addition, patients having mid-face augmentation should avoid blowing their noses for the first week after surgery.

The skin tapes placed after chin augmentation are removed at 5–6 days. After either chin or mid-face augmentation, the patient may be seen socially after a week although a little swelling may still be present and the smile may still be "a little stiff" for a few more days.

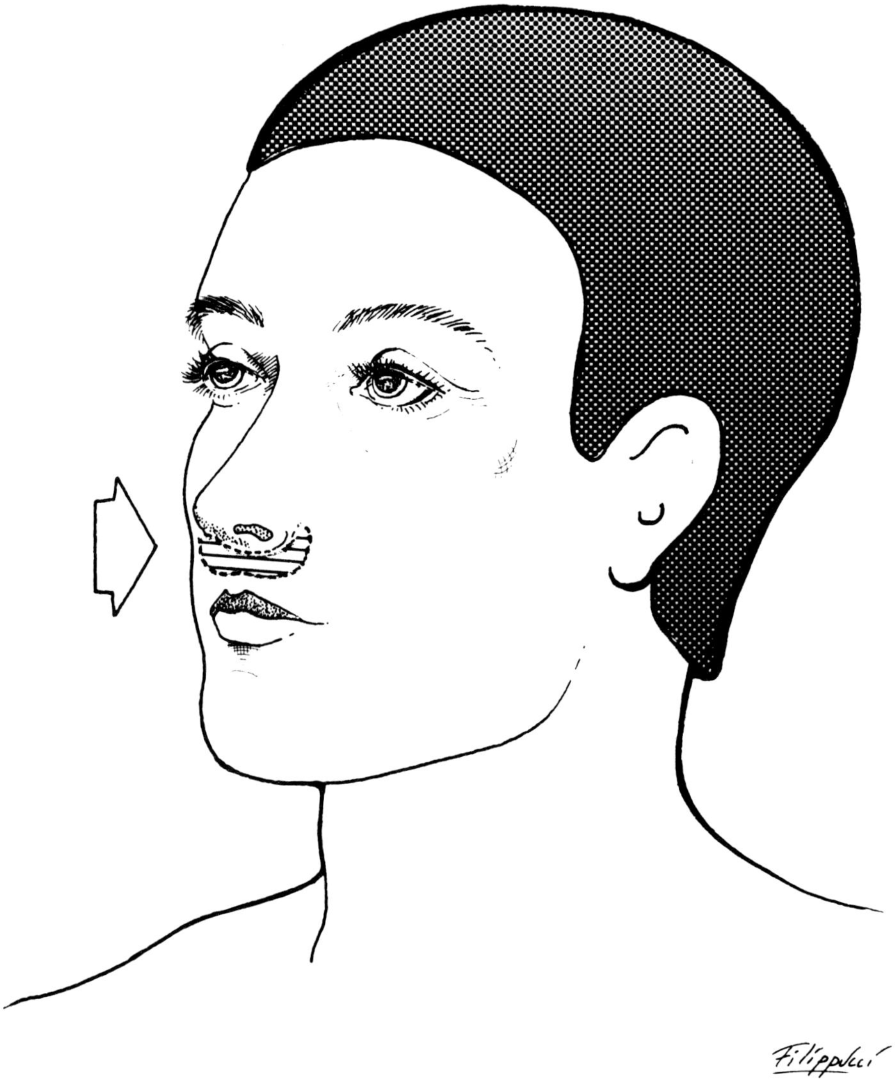

FIGURE 11: The arrow illustrates the location and shape of the implant for mid-face *(maxillary)* augmentation.

Although it usually has little effect, direct sunlight should be avoided for 3 weeks postoperatively unless a sunblock is used because it has the potential for increasing and prolonging any residual swelling. The face should be washed gently for the first 2 weeks to avoid possible movement of the implants. Contact sports should be avoided for 3 weeks for the same reason.

PRECAUTIONS AND POTENTIAL PROBLEMS

Asymmetry may rarely result from a slight slipping of one of the implants in the first few days. Fortunately this can usually be solved by gentle manipulation and re-taping for a few more days; occasionally an implant must be surgically repositioned. This is why the patient *must* allow the tapes to remain in position after chin augmentation for at least 5 days. Fortunately both chin and midface implants rarely slip since they are carved to fit a bony prominence.

Rarely in chin or mid-face augmentation, one of the muscles which move the lip may be bruised. This will result in a *temporarily asymmetric smile*. The smile always returns to normal in a week or two.

Infection occurs very rarely since the solid silicon implants are well-tolerated. However, suitable antibiotics would be used to treat it and the implant might have to be removed in a severe case.

FINISHING TOUCHES

If the chin is somewhat "pointy" in addition to being receded, I will shape the implant to round out the jawline by sculpting an implant with more fullness on the sides than in front. While the chin is being augmented to improve the profile, it may, as was illustrated in the case history, be appropriate to remove any nasal hump present by concurrent *rhinoplasty* (see **Photos 9**, **10** and **11**).

If there is extra fat beneath the chin, it may be advantageous to perform a *submental lipectomy* while placing the chin implant. In older patients, sometimes *cheeklift* or *facelift* may be required to further improve the jaw and neckline.

In some patients with pointy or receded chins, a second set of wrinkles appear from the corners of the mouth to the chin. One of my patients referred to these as "Howdy Dowdy lines". In addition to a specially-sculpted chin implant, *collagen injections* may help in the elimination of these lines.

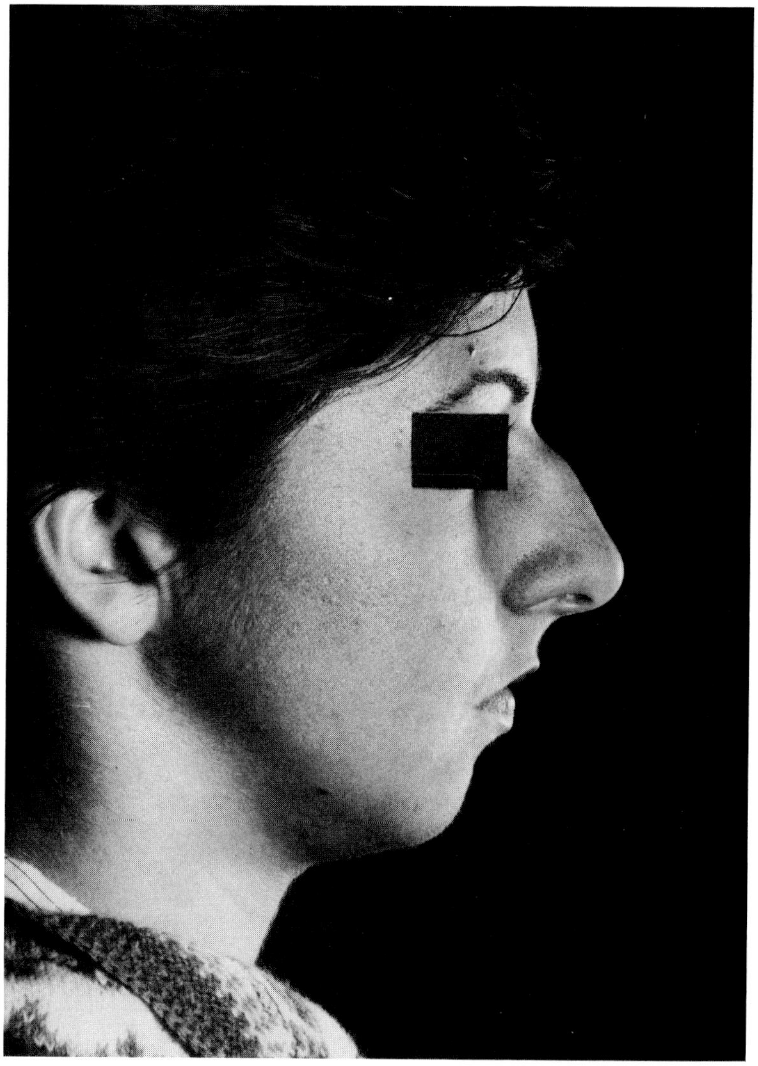

PHOTO 9: A patient with a nasal hump, short upper lip and receding chin.

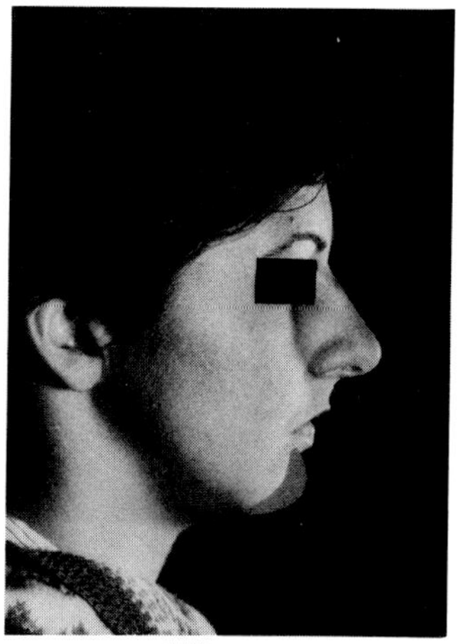

PHOTO 10: Preoperative sketch showing planned chin augmentation and nasal reduction.

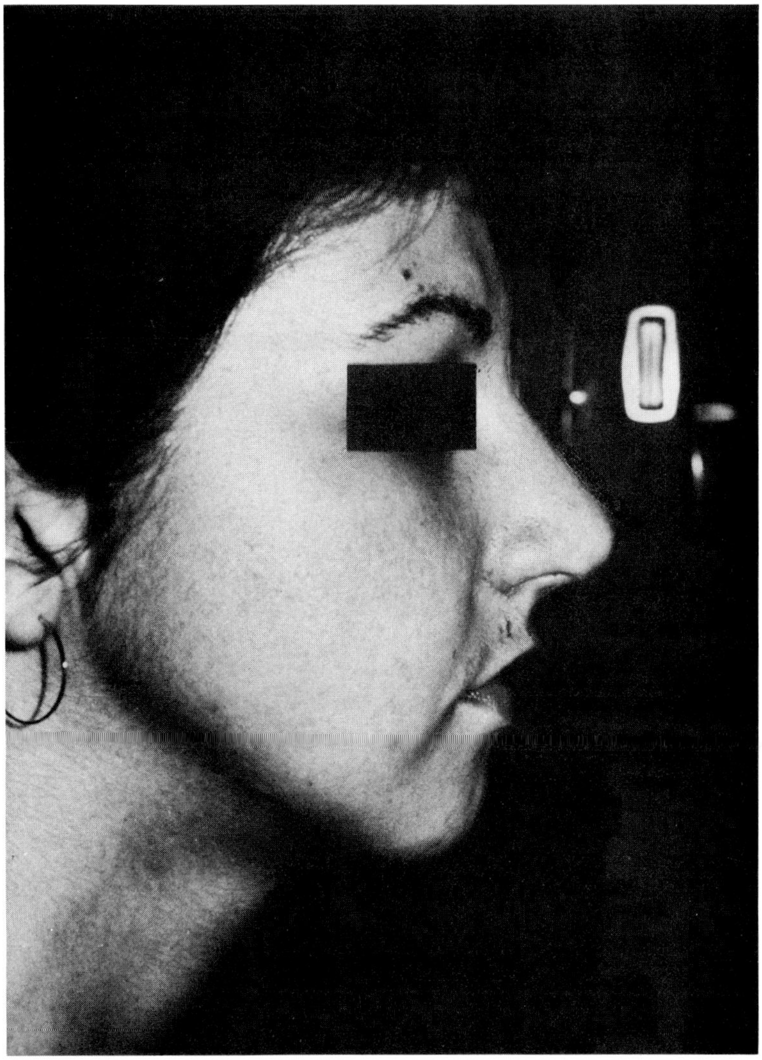

PHOTO 11: Same patient following *rhinoplasty* and chin augmentation.

If the mid-face is being made more prominent, it may also be desireable to perform a *rhinoplasty* to give even more projection to the nose and correct any nasal bulbousness or tip droop at the same time. It is also possible to further correct the deep hollows that occur beneath and along side of the nostrils in these patients with *collagen injections*.

It is not uncommon for the cheek bones to be somewhat "invisible" in those with "dish-face" deformity. *Cheek augmentation*, which is discussed in the next chapter, may very much enhance the surgical results in these patients.

* * *

CHAPTER 21

The High Fashion Look through Cheek Implants

Many patients with long and narrow faces or those with full cheeks and "invisible" cheek bones long for the dramatic effect of "high" cheek bones. The fashion magazines are replete with photographs of male and female models from the Midwest or Nordic heritage who possess the "high-fashion look." This look is readily obtainable through a simple office procedure.

Solid silicon implants may be shaped to achieve the desired result and be inserted through the mouth to add prominence and projection to patient's own cheek bones. If the patient has an unusual face, I will occasionally make a *moulage* (clay-like model) and fabricate a custom-made implant from this fast-setting plaster. More usually, I will carve a silicon implant at the operating room table to achieve the desired result.

The effect of these implants is dramatic; the patient's face can be either subtlely or radically changed. The surgeon can literally sculpt faces to order. If only cheek augmentation is being performed, I will perform this *malar augmentation* through the mouth. If lower lids, cheek or facelift is being performed, I will use one of these routes for implant insertion instead.

A nice side benefit of *malar augmentation* is that the hollows beneath the lower lids *(nasojugal folds)* are usually softened by this procedure without any direct surgical attention. There is usually significant swelling but little bruising. This generally subsides by the end of a week. The sutures within

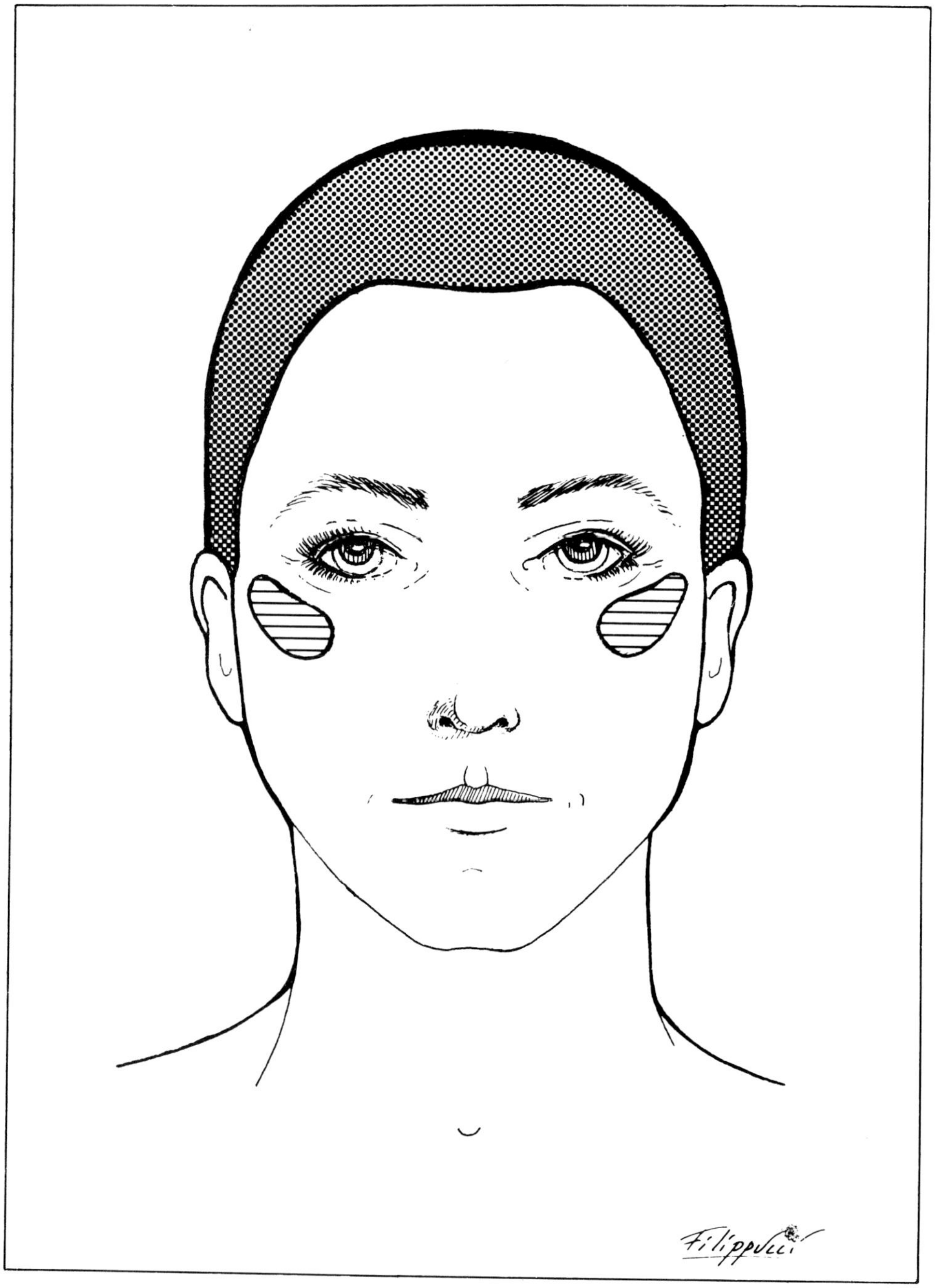

FIGURE 12: The proper placement of implants to render the cheekbones more prominent is shown *(malar augmentation)*.

the mouth dissolve and need not be removed. Performed as a solitary procedure, cheek augmentation only requires one week before the patient is seen socially. As an ancillary procedure to face or eyelid lift, it does not add to the time required for convalescence.

A fluid diet is suggested for the first postoperative day and a soft diet for the following day so that chewing can be avoided. I always prescribe broad-spectrum antibiotics since it is difficult to "sterilize" the mouth.

CASE HISTORY

P.N. was a very slender 45-year-old housewife with a long, narrow face. For years she had longed for more prominent cheek bones and deeply shadowed her cheeks to imitate this effect. She finally decided to consult a Plastic Surgeon to see if something could be done. She desired a very striking and dramatic look and would not be satisfied with a subtle change.

Under local anaesthesia in the office, implants were carved to achieve the desired effect and inserted through her mouth. The patient was not only ecstatic that her dream had been achieved so simply, but was also pleased that the slight hollows beneath her lower lids had also been eliminated.

PREPARATION

The usual *Vitamin K and C are prescribed* while *Vitamin E and aspirin-containing products are avoided for 2 weeks preoperatively. Medical Photographs* are essential for preoperative planning; specific views are included to illustrate the cheek bones. *Xrays* may occasionally be required to elucidate unusual conditions.

The face is washed with *Phisohex®*, the teeth are brushed, and the mouth rinsed with hydrogen peroxide and Listerine® on the morning of surgery. No make-up, contacts or false eyelashes are worn. If the patient wears dentures, these should be worn to the office. Several types very much influence the upper lip and cheek area.

THE PROCEDURE

Before proceeding with surgery, I made sketches upon the patient's face to establish the proper location and axis of the implant upon the patient's own cheek bones. This location is related to the ear canal and the corners of the eyes and mouth to achieve proper symmetry.

After preliminary sedation and intravenous relaxants, the *mucosa* (lining of the mouth) above the upper premolars is injected with local anesthetic. Through this numb area, a slightly longer needle is used to numb the cheek.

A small incision is made in the numbed area, in the groove between the gum and cheek, above the premolars and the bottom border of the cheek bone is immediately accessible. The overlying muscle and skin is raised from the cheek bone without need for cutting. Through this "keyhole", the implant is inserted; it may be removed and re-carved several times before I am satisfied (see **Fig. 12**). When I am certain that the desired effect has been achieved, I will carve a matching implant and insert it on the other side.

Any bleeding is controlled with electrocautery. The *mucosa* is sewn with individual sutures that dissolve in 2 to 3 weeks. Elastic tapes are placed upon the patient's cheeks to keep the implant well-approximated to the skin and underlying cheek bone. These are allowed to remain in place for 5–6 days and are crucial to the final result.

RECUPERATION

The patient will take a fluid diet for the evening of surgery. The following day a soft diet is permitted. The upper teeth should be brushed gently and the mouth rinsed with a mix of salt water and hydrogen peroxide after meals and at bedtime for the first 3 days. It is recommended that the patient try to sleep flat on his or her back rather than on either side for the first week. A broad-spectrum antibiotic, generally *Keflex*®, is prescribed since the mouth cannot be rendered totally free of germs.

The skin tapes placed after cheek augmentation are removed at 5–6 days. The patient may be seen socially after a week although a little swelling may still be present and the smile may still be "a little stiff" for a few more days.

Although it usually has little effect, direct sunlight should be avoided for 3 weeks post-operatively unless a sunblock is used because it has the potential for increasing and prolonging any residual swelling. The face should be washed gently for the first 2 weeks to avoid possible movement of the implants. Contact spots should be avoided for 3 weeks for the same reason. Modest cheek augmentation is illustrated in **Photos 12** and **13**.

PRECAUTIONS AND POTENTIAL PROBLEMS

Asymmetry may sometimes result from a slight slipping of one of the cheek implants in the first few days. Fortunately this can usually be solved by gentle manipulation and re-taping for a few more days; occasionally an implant must be surgically repositioned. This is why the patient *must* allow the tapes to remain in position for at least 5 days.

Rarely in cheek augmentation, one of the muscles which lift the corner of the mouth may be bruised. This will result in a *temporarily asymmetric smile.* The smile always returns to normal in a week or two.

Infection occurs very rarely since the solid silicon implants are well-tolerated. However, suitable antibiotics would be used to treat it and the implants might have to be removed in a severe case.

FINISHING TOUCHES

In patients undergoing cheek augmentation, total correction of any hollows beneath the lower lids may be achieved by concurrent *lower eyelid lift.* It may also be desireable to *defat the cheeks* of a round-faced individual to enhance the effect of cheek bone augmentation. It is also possible to concurrently round out a pointy chin in a long-faced individual with a suitably-carved *chin implant.*

Since the cheek skin tends to fall with aging, leaving thinner skin over the cheek bones, *cheek or facelift* may be indicated to correct this problem and further improve the patient's appearance along with cheek augmentation. Since cheek implants frequently have the side benefit that the laughline creases *(nasolabial folds)* are softened, *collagen injections* may be employed to further enhance this effect.

Since the width of the face, as determined by the cheek bones, partially determines whether a nose looks broad or bulbous, it may be desireable to specifically treat any bulbousness of the nasal tip or broadness of the nasal bridge with *rhinoplasty* to further improve the appearance in suitable patients undergoing cheek augmentation.

* * *

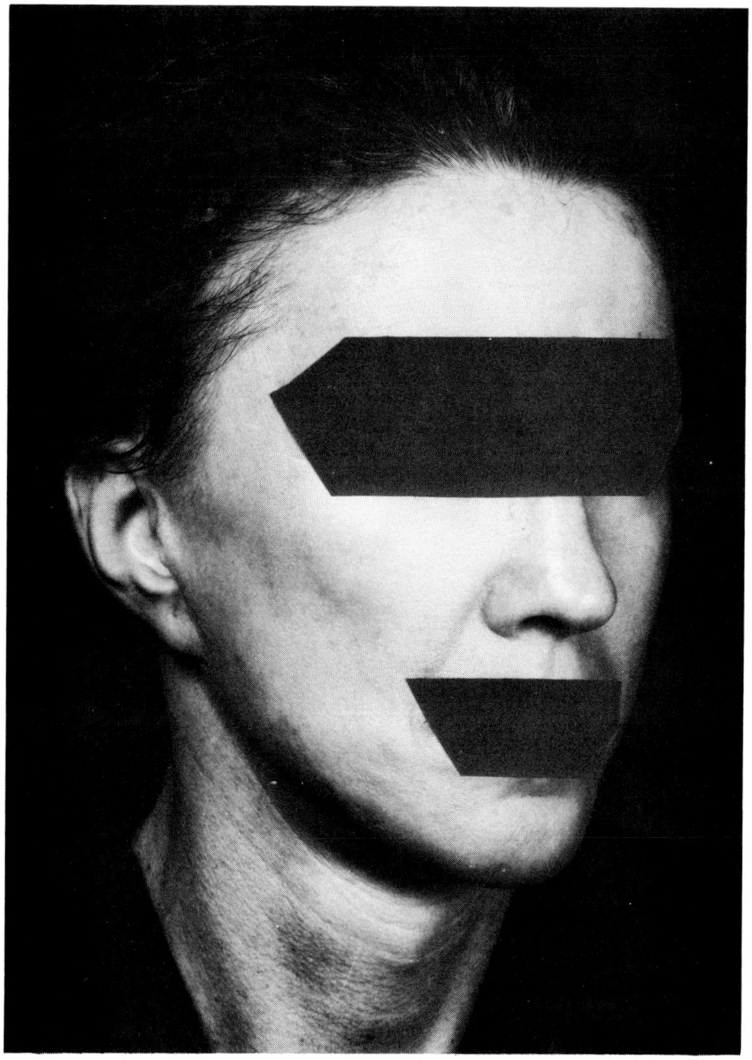

PHOTO 12: A patient without very prominent cheek bones.

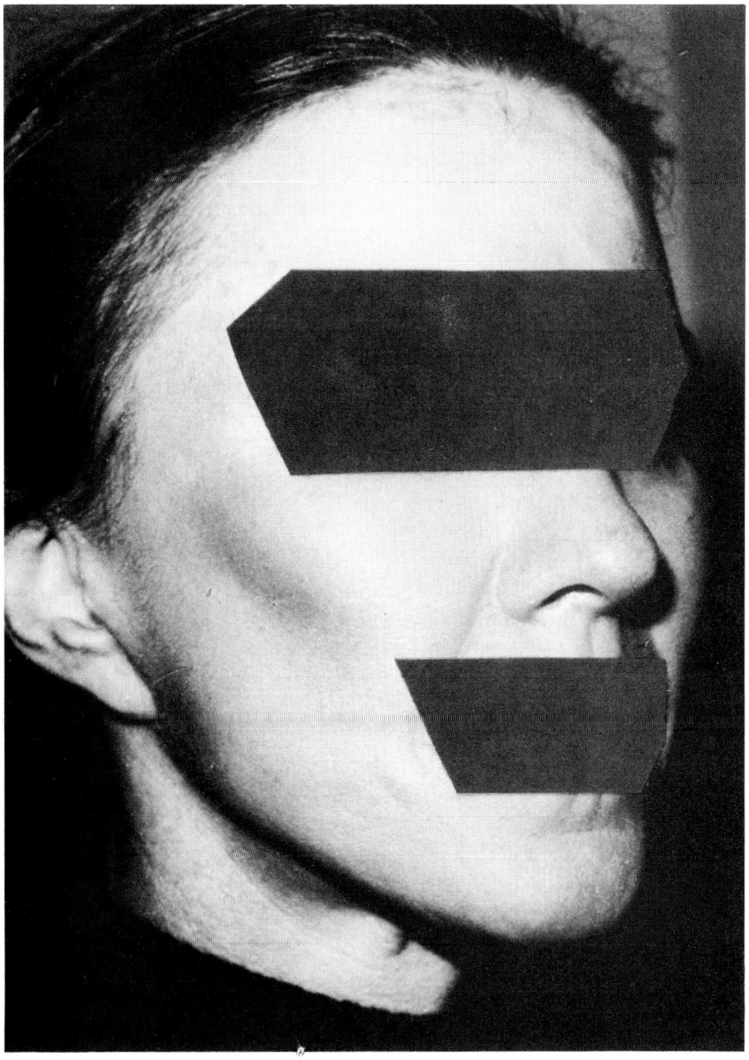

PHOTO 13: The same patient after *malar augmentation*.

CHAPTER 22

A Nose Sculpted for Your Face

The nose is the most prominent feature on the face. The width of the nasal bridge influences the appearance of the eyes and the length of the nose affects the perceptual and actual length of the upper lip. Its projection relates to the forehead and chin in what should be a harmonious relationship. The relation of the fleshy mid-portion *(columnella)* and nostrils *(alae)* helps to determine the expression of the face. The broadness of the nasal bridge determines "how large the eyes are"; people with sunken and broad nasal bridges (like a prize fighter's) give a "stupid" appearance.

The nose is one of the areas of the body where surgery can be performed under local anesthesia with a minimum of risk; results can be maximally visible with as marked or subtle alteration of the patient's appearance as desired. The surgery is a brief, relatively painless procedure on surface anatomy; as such *rhinoplasty* is one of the most frequently requested and discussed plastic surgical procedures, and the operation may be sought for correction of breathing difficulties, asymmetries or widening from old injuries, or ethnic heritage.

The ideal time of intervention on the nose is after it has achieved most of its adult growth, which is in adolescent years, preferably before the later years of dating in high school. It must be remembered that a good result is one which satisfies the patient; the patient and surgeon must discuss in detail the goals and expectations of the procedure. Altered sketches and pre-

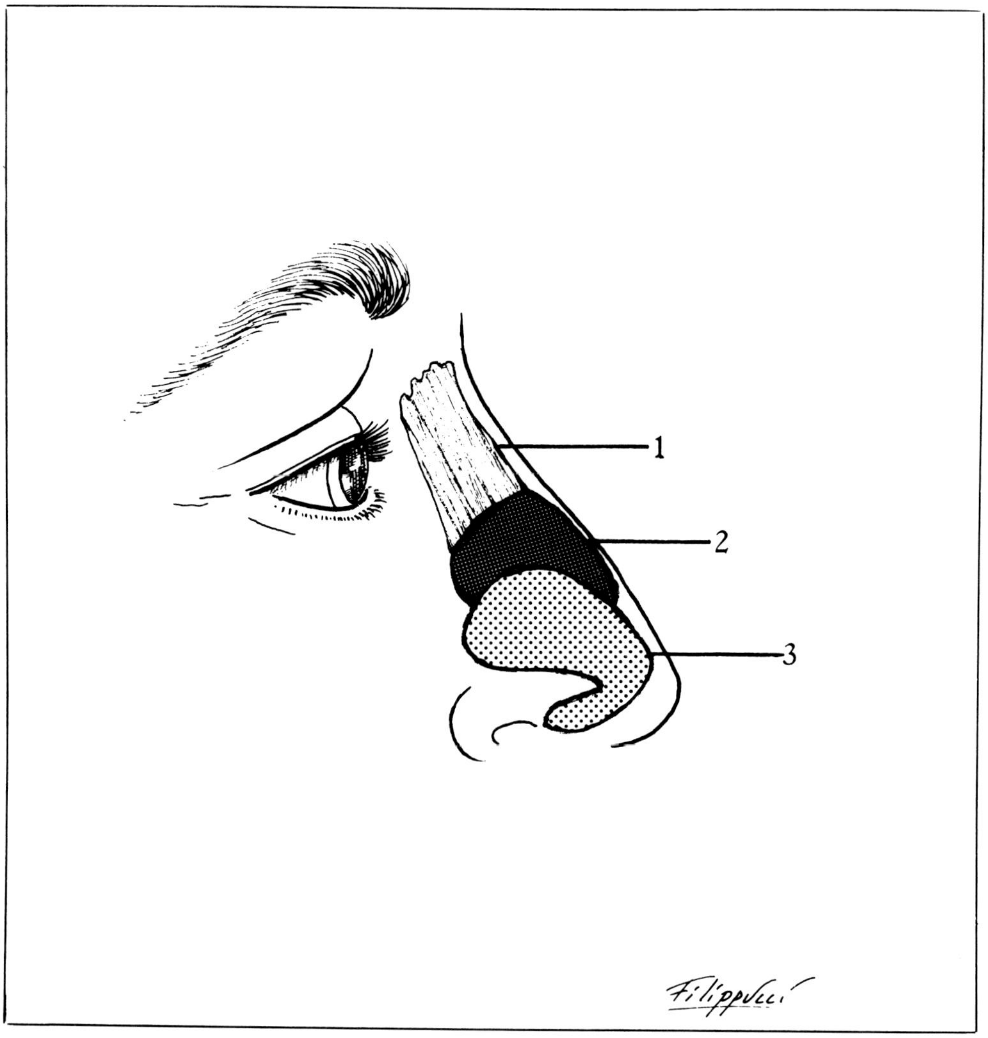

FIGURE 13: Normal nasal anatomy: 1—nasal bone; 2—*quadrangular cartilage*; 3—*alar cartilage*. (Reprinted from *The Kindest Cut*.)

operative photographs may help indicate to the patient what the surgeon is striving for, and to the surgeon, what the patient desires. Naturally, by virtue of the uncontrollable factors related to individual healing, the preoperative sketches cannot show guaranteed results. Nevertheless, preoperative evaluation with proper medical photographs is imperative for its value in communication of patient's desires and surgeon's intents, and its importance in preoperative planning and objective postoperative evaluation and comparison. Examination of carefully taken preoperative photographs may also be helpful in illustrating whether additional procedures may be desireable, such as *augmentation mentoplasty*, to make the chin more prominent.

The upper portion of the nose is supported by paired nasal bones and the bony septum. The lower portion is supported by two sets of paired cartilages and the cartilaginous portion of the septum (see **Fig. 13**). Both portions are contained within an adherent skin envelope. The bony portions of the nose may be altered with great predictability, but there is much variability in individual healing with regard to correction of the soft portions of the nose, namely the cartilage and the redraping of the skin over the altered skeleton in the manner of a deflating balloon. Older, sun-damaged, oily or thick skin is inferior in its ability to redrape and shrink. Marked alteration of the size of the nasal skeleton is occasionally accompanied by very slow or incomplete redraping of the skin in these individuals; secondary procedures using either cartilage grafts to "take up" the extra skin or external incisions (in addition to the usual internal, non-visible incisions commonly used for nasal surgery) may be indicated to obtain optimal results. Younger patients or older patients requiring lesser changes are generally better candidates because of the greater elasticity of their skin and its better ability to redrape.

Blacks or Orientals who desire to have their noses changed to a more Caucasian type of nose may have this done surgically. The original anatomy is one of a depressed bridge or *saddle* nose, and wide, flaring nostrils. The saddle nose may be corrected with a silastic implant, straightening the nasal profile and adding to tip projection. The nostrils may be narrowed and their thickness reduced. Pre- and postoperative care is the same as for conventional *rhinoplasty*, and this procedure may be carried out in the office or hospital under local anesthesia.

The patient desiring *rhinoplasty* should set aside a week and expect to cover some lower eyelid brusing with make-up during the second week if appearing socially. The procedure takes about one hour and is generally performed under local anesthesia in the office. A molded nasal splint is placed at the end of the procedure and is allowed to remain in position for one week.

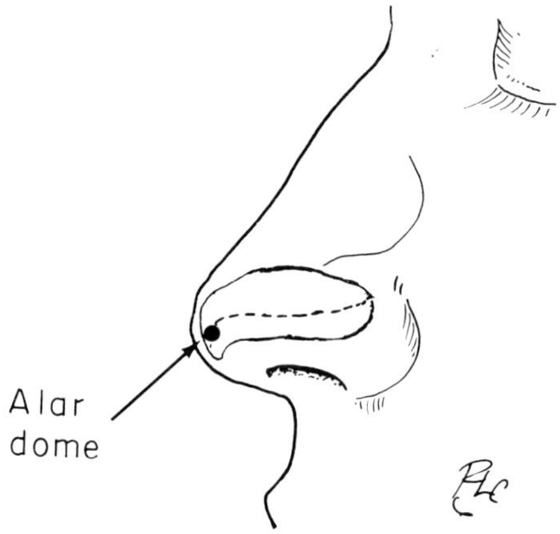

FIGURE 14: The alar cartilage is usually responsible for bulbous nasal tips. The most projecting portion of each of the paired alar cartilages is referred to as the *alar dome*. By removing "extra" alar cartilage (that above the dashed line), the tip can be refined and its projection decreased. (Adapted from "An Aid to Tailoring the Alar Cartilages in Tip Rhinoplasty", R.L. Cucin, *Plastic and Reconstructive Surgery* 65:828.)

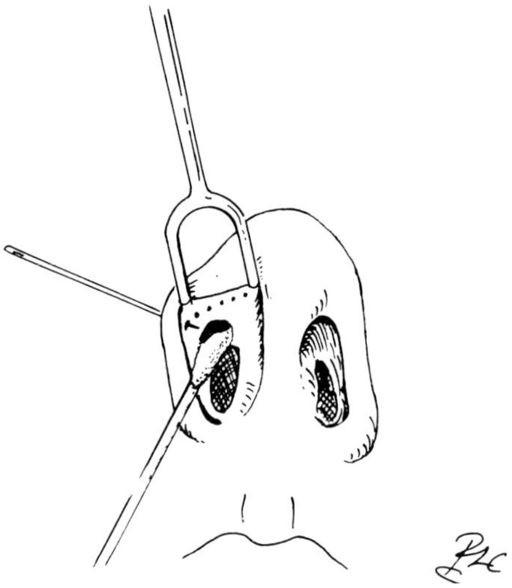

FIGURE 15: The individualized pattern of cartilage removed to achieve the desired effect is first sketched on the outside of the nose; it is then transferred internally by transfixion with fine needles, moistening their tips with vital dye, and withdrawing them. Precise placement of the internal incision results. (Adapted from "An Aid to Tailoring the Alar Cartilages in Tip Rhinoplasty", R.L. Cucin, *Plastic and Reconstructive Surgery* 65:828.)

CASE HISTORY

E.T. was an attractive cocktail waitress from the Bronx who had a slight nasal hump and slightly bulbous nasal tip. After having her teeth bonded to give her an attractive smile, she wanted to finish the job by improving the appearance of her nose.

Under local anesthesia in the office, her nasal hump was shaved and the nasal tip refined. She was very pleased with the refined look to her nose and worked diligently afterwards to drop her "Bronx accent" in keeping with the improvements in her appearance.

PREPARATION

Because of the heavy supplementary medication usually employed, the patient undergoing *rhinoplasty* is required to avoid eating after midnight the night before surgery, even though the operation is customarily performed under local. *Vitamin K and Vitamin C are prescribed before surgery* to help promote ideal healing and to minimize bruising. Preparation of the skin of the face with *Phisohex*® is suggested to eliminate troublesome bacteria even prior to surgical scrubbing of the operative field. *Aspirin, aspirin-containing products and Vitamin E should be avoided for two weeks before surgery* because they increase bleeding and bruising. The procedure may be performed in the office on an outpatient basis.

Medical Photographs are essential to preoperative planning. I will usually have a second consultation with patients after I have sketched the planned procedure upon matted profile photographs (see **Photos 10, 15, 18** and **27**). This helps me to communicate my intentions and to better understand the patient's desires. It also serves to help point out those individuals in whom surgical results might be enhanced by a simultaneous chin augmentation.

THE PROCEDURE

Just prior to surgery, the patient is prepared with several injections for sedation; an intravenous is inserted and additional sedation is administered as necessary. Cotton-tipped applicators dipped in anesthetizing solution are placed within the nose to numb the inside lining.

I will first make sketches on the outside of the nose at the level of hump removal. Then I will make markings at the sites of tip refinement and narrowing and transfer these to the inside of the nose (see **Figs. 14** and **15**). This allows a very precise and individualized tailoring of the patient's *alar cartilages*, the lower paired cartilages which determine the shape, breadth and projection of the tip of the nose. By this method the "pinched" nostril look so common a decade ago is avoided.

Meanwhile the inner lining of the nose has become numb; now, local anesthetic solution is injected and constitutes the only discomfort the patient will feel throughout the procedure. First, the cartilages of the tip are refined and a "droopy tip" is lifted. Then the paired cartilages of the mid-portion of the nose *(quadrangular cartilages)* are lowered and shortened in accordance with the planned profile. Lastly, the bony nasal hump is removed and the bones repositioned to effect any desired narrowing. The key words during all four steps of the procedure are *natural* and *conservatism.* It is much easier to shave off a little more hump than replace it after too much has been removed—although this can be done too. I much prefer a natural straight nose to a markedly "turned up" or retrousse nose. A good *rhinoplasty* result is a nose which does *not* look "done"!

Although I can usually anticipate the need for this preoperatively, it is at the final point in surgery when I look at the nostrils and decide if it would be flattering to make them somewhat smaller or thinner with *Weir resections.* Tapes are then applied to the skin and a molded plaster of Paris splint applied. A loose nasal packing is placed in each nostril.

RECUPERATION

Patients are generally rather fatigued the rest of the day and will usually sleep off the medication. Iced compresses to your eyelids for the first 72 hours will minimize the bruising and swelling from the bony alteration. A soft diet which requires little chewing is suggested for the evening of surgery.

On the following morning, the nasal packing is removed unless there has been extensive septal surgery; 6 days later the split is removed. The splint and tapes are critically important for maintaining the direct application of the skin to the newly altered nasal skeleton and they are necessary for achievement of the final desired result.

Bruising customarily persists for 10–14 days with black and blue marks around the eyelids gradually resorbing. These can be covered with make-up during the second week. By two weeks the patient is ready to appear socially.

It is best to avoid wearing eyeglasses for the first three weeks to prevent pressure on the nasal bridge; if needed, they may be taped to the forehead to keep them off the newly realigned nasal bones. Special glasses have been developed for this purpose and I provide them for patients requiring them. Contact sports should be avoided for the first six weeks, although non-contact sports such as tennis or jogging may be resumed after three weeks.

Some degree of swelling persists from weeks to months as the nasal contour improves slowly and steadily over the following year until it has achieved its final appearance. The sun exacerbates any swelling present and should be avoided for the first 4 weeks unless a sunblock is used. **Photos 14–28** show postoperative results.

PRECAUTIONS AND POTENTIAL PROBLEMS

As with any facial surgery, *bleeding* may rarely occur during the postoperative period. Generally a few days of nasal packing are the only treatment required. The nasal splint must be allowed to remain on while the packing is in place so the nasal skeleton will not be widened.

If too much has been asked of the skin, if it has been asked to shrink beyond its capacity in the correction of a large hump or bulbous tip, *incomplete redraping* may occur. This can present as a *supratip* deformity which is a rise in the lower one-third of the nasal profile. It can also present as a slightly droopy tip. Both of these conditions are easily corrected, generally at the end of a year, by which time the skin will have shrunken about 85% to 95% as much as it will. In most cases a small cartilage graft *(tip graft)* can be obtained from a non-supportative portion of the nasal septum and used to add definition, lift if required, and "take up the slack" of any skin redundancy. I will always inform those few patients in whom I think it likely that this later, *secondary rhinoplasty* might be valuable in obtaining the best possible results (see **Photos 29** and **30**).

Minor *asymmetry* is a possibility in all nasal surgery, both during the course of cartilage resection and by possibly "unmasking" a previously undiagnosed septal deviation. The possibility of this happening is very much reduced by careful preoperative examination and the technique of sketched resection as described in the operative procedure. Cartilage grafts or collagen injections can both be used to treat this problem if it should occur.

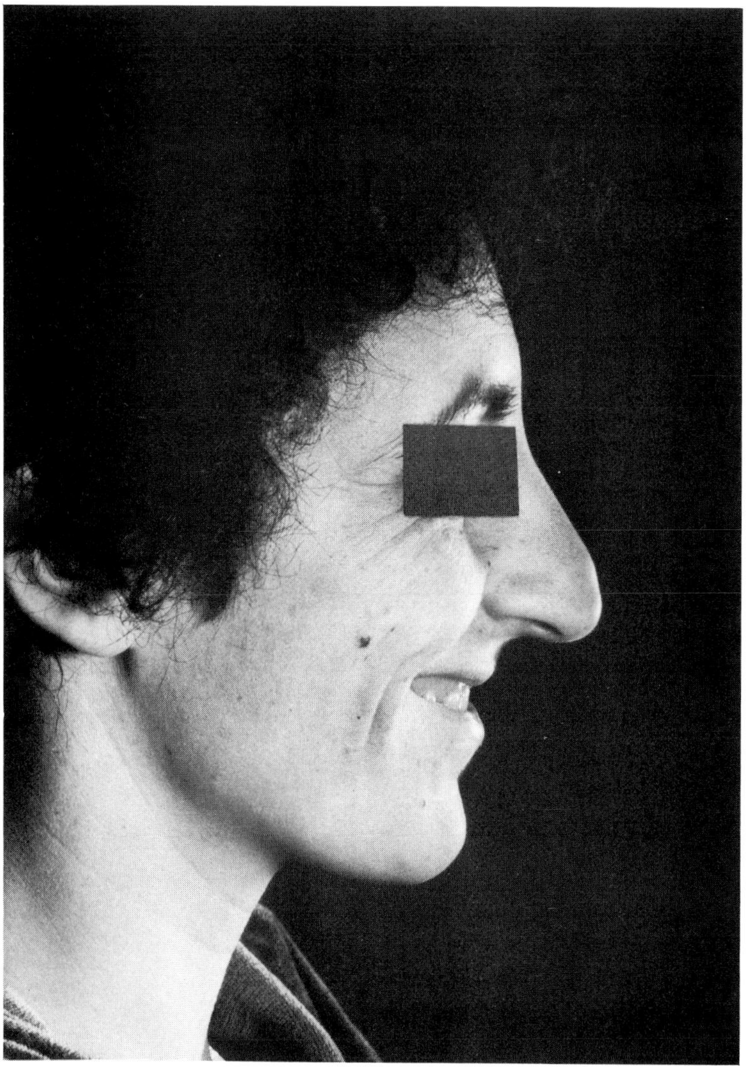

PHOTO 14: A patient with a large, droopy nose.

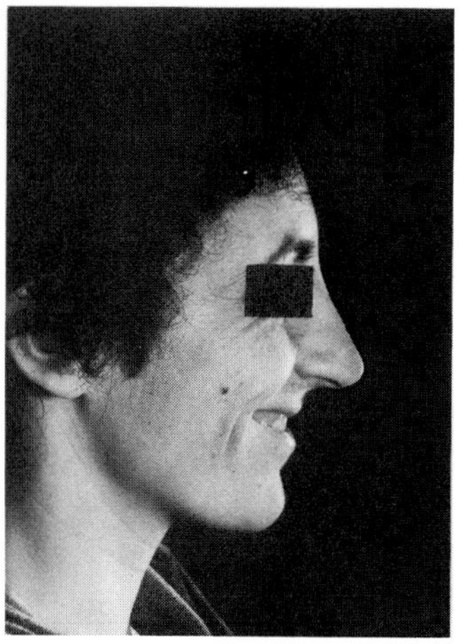

PHOTO 15: The preoperative sketch of planned nasal reduction.

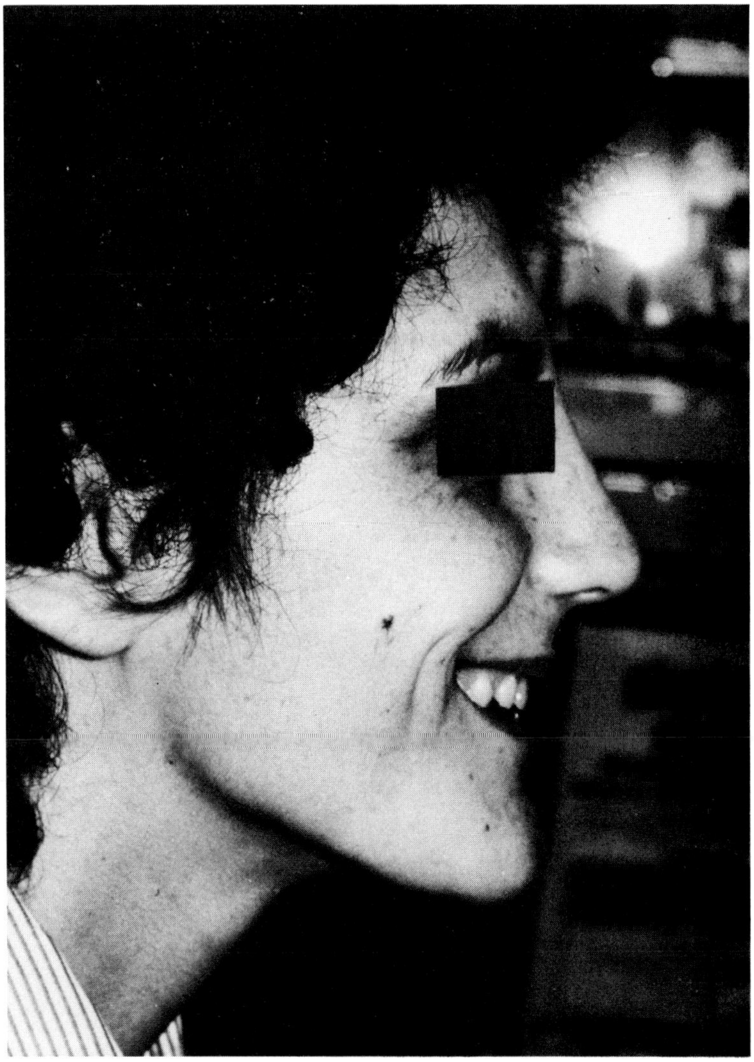

PHOTO 16: The same patient after nasal reduction.

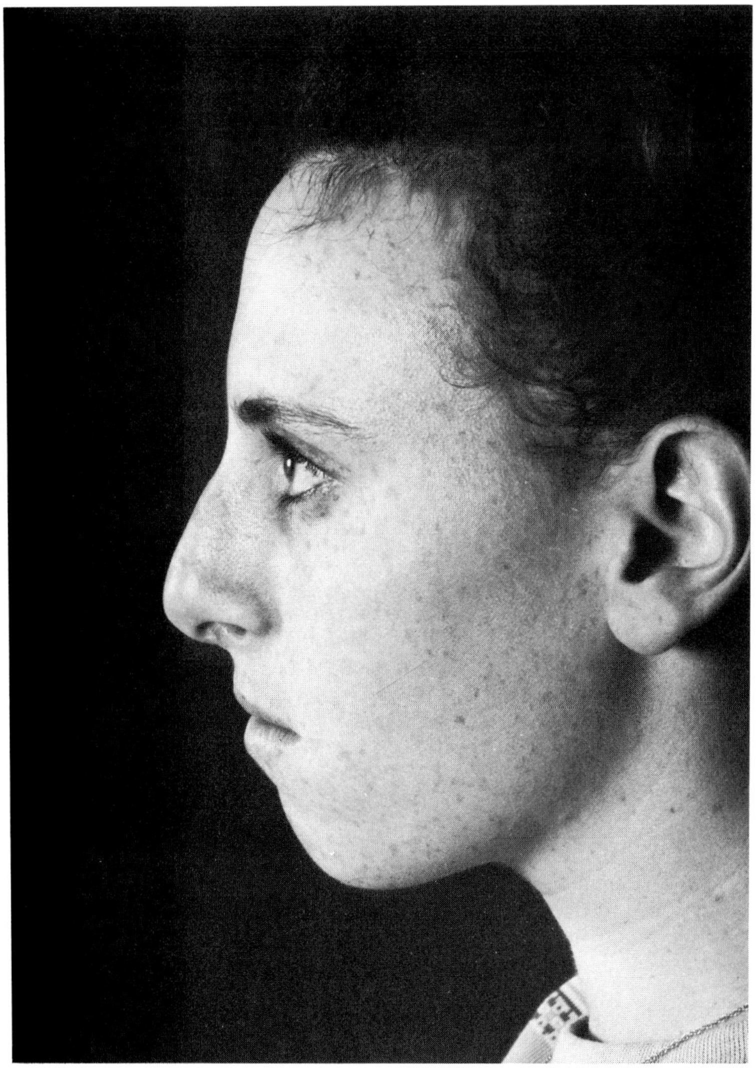

PHOTO 17: A patient with a nasal hump and receding chin.

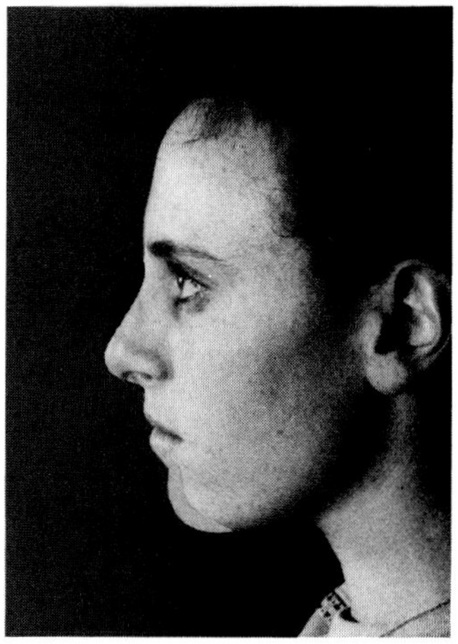

PHOTO 18: The preoperative sketch of planned nasal reduction and chin augmentation.

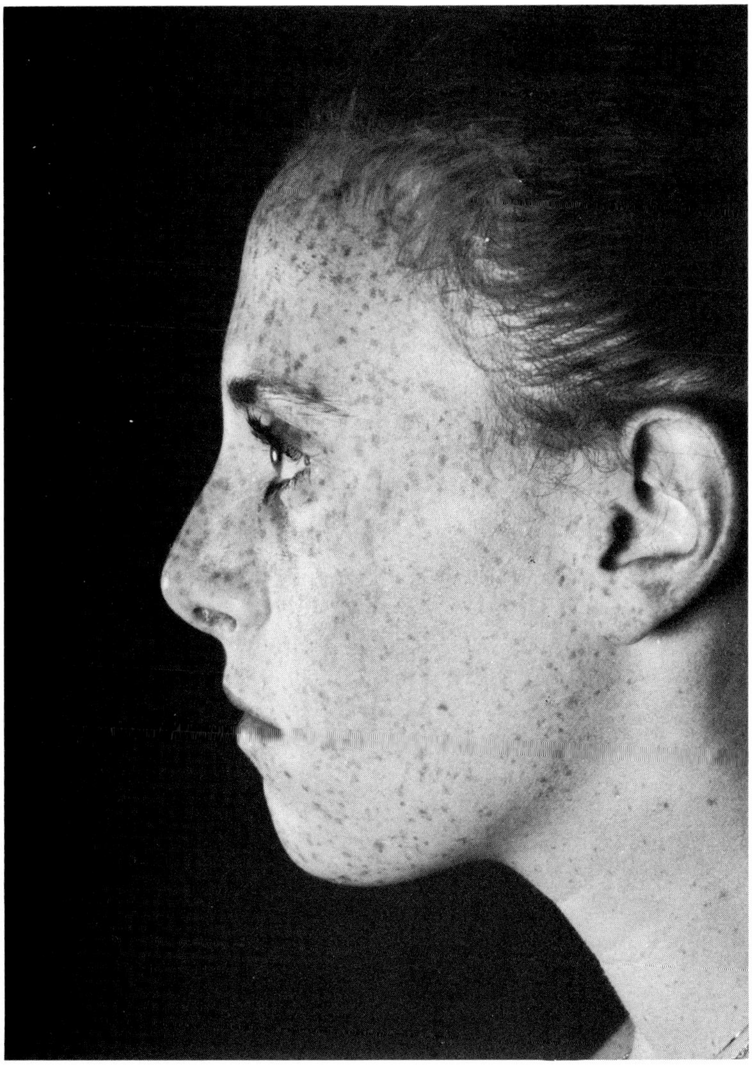

PHOTO 19: The same patient after *rhinoplasty* and chin augmentation. (The prominence of the patient's freckles after unscreened Summer-sun exposure demonstrates the sun's effect in making these freckles more noticeable.)

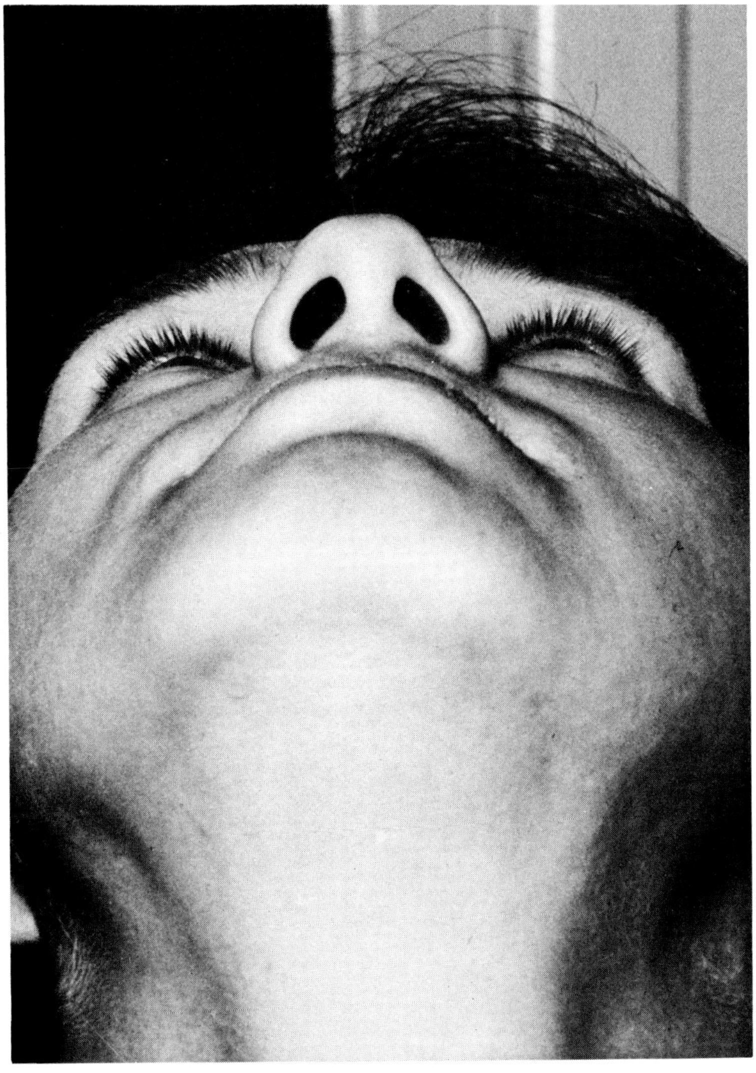

PHOTO 20: "Worm's eye" view of a patient with a bulbous *(bifid)* nasal tip.

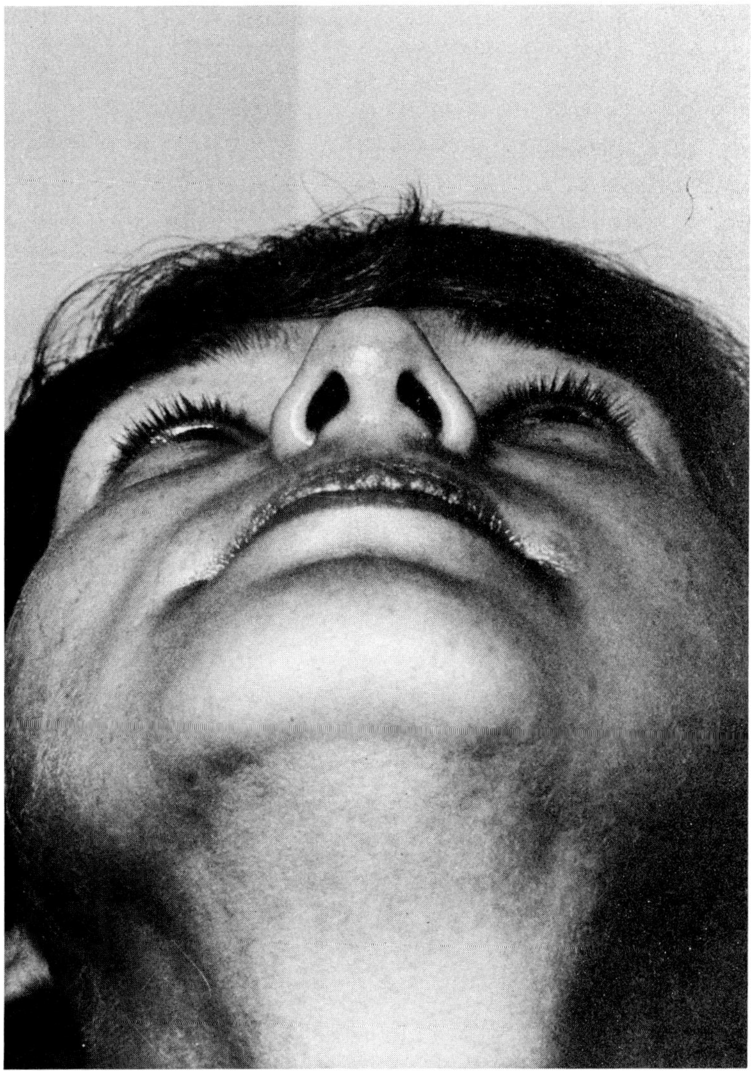

PHOTO 21: The same patient after *tip rhinoplasty*.

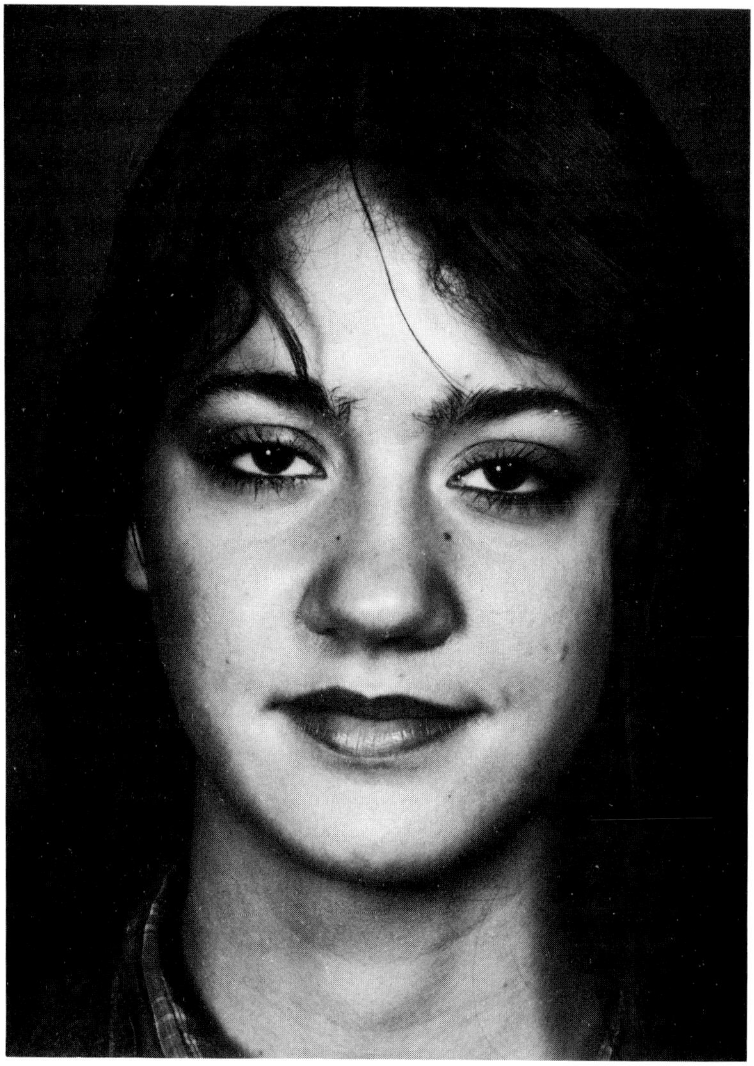

PHOTO 22: A patient with a broad nasal tip.

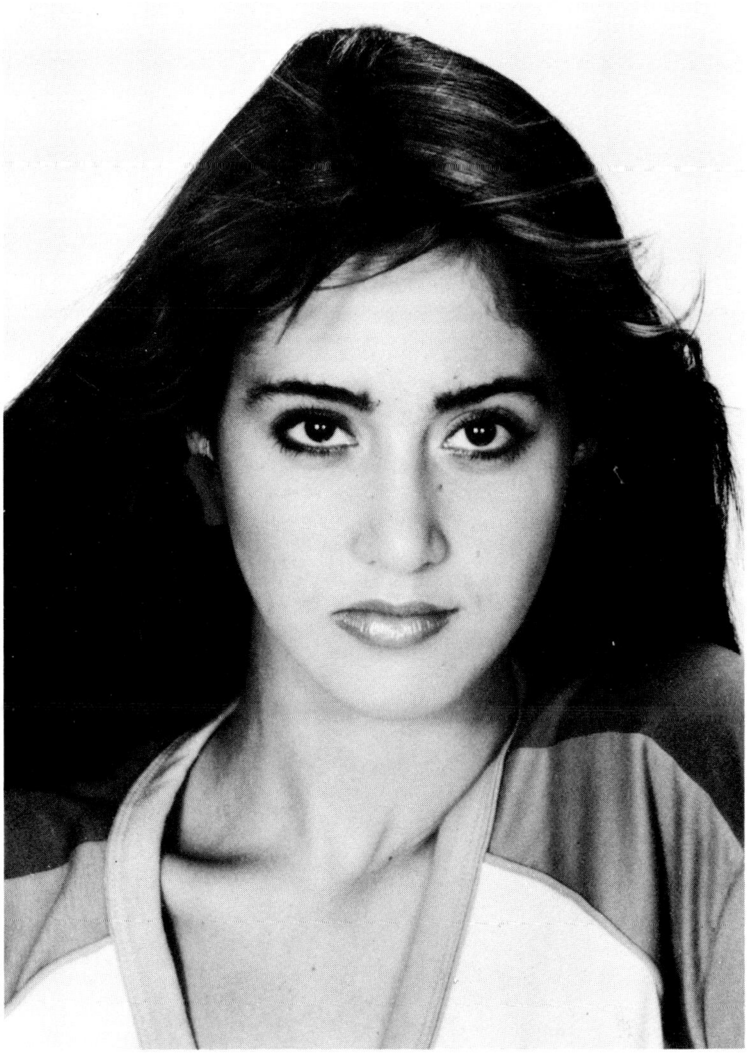

PHOTO 23: The same patient after *rhinoplasty*.

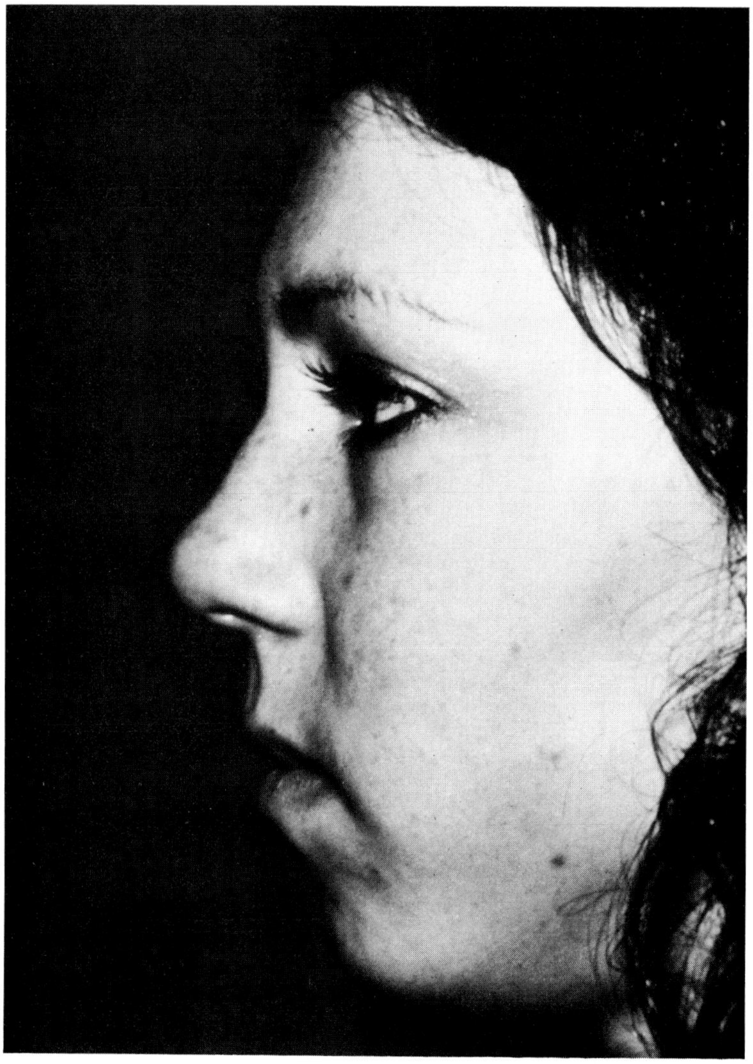

PHOTO 24: A patient with a small nasal hump, bulbous tip and receding chin.

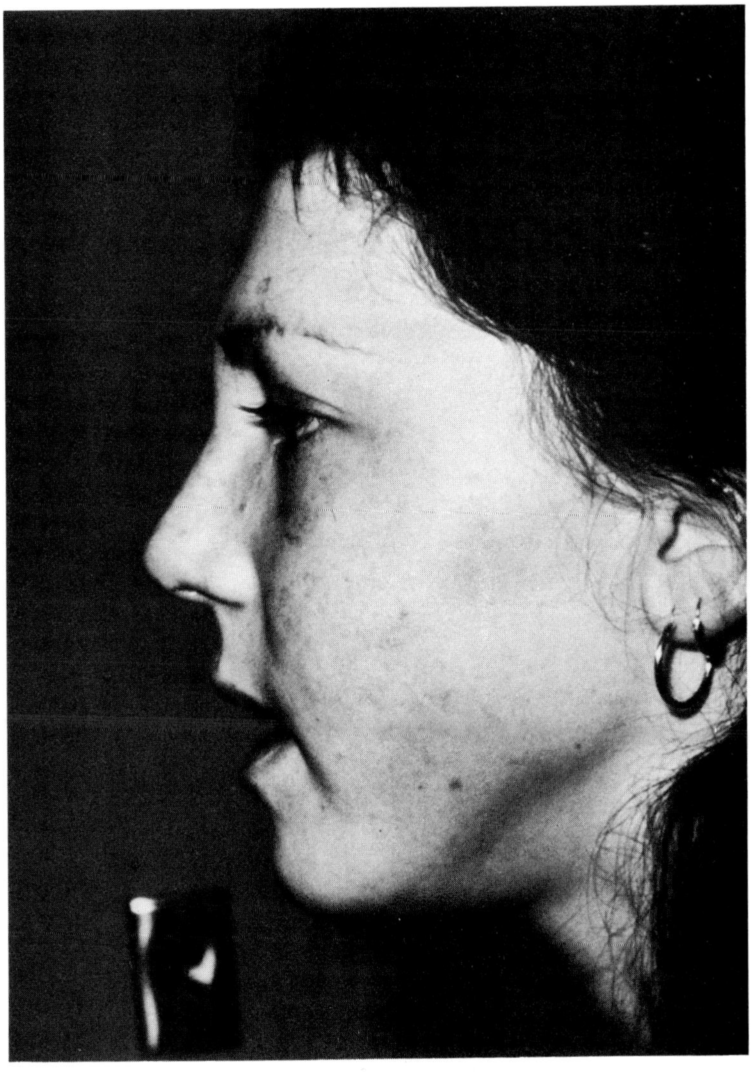

PHOTO 25: The same patient after a "finesse" *rhinoplasty* and chin augmentation.

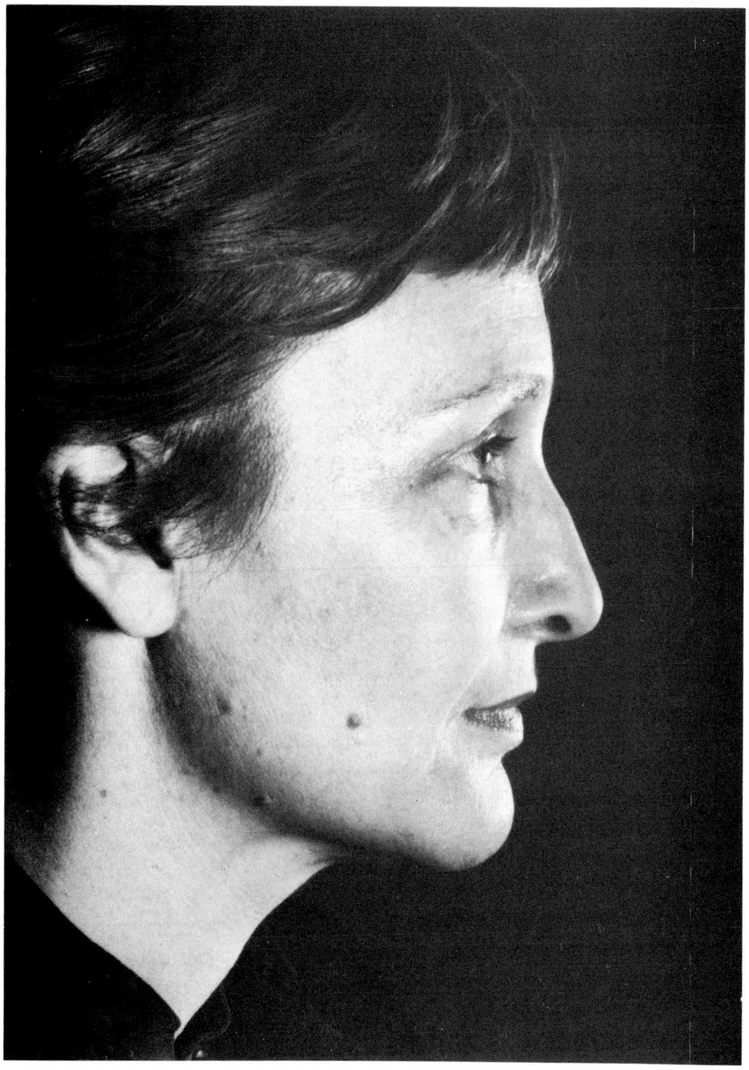

PHOTO 26: A patient with a small nasal hump and slight "tip droop" giving her a stern, slightly older appearance.

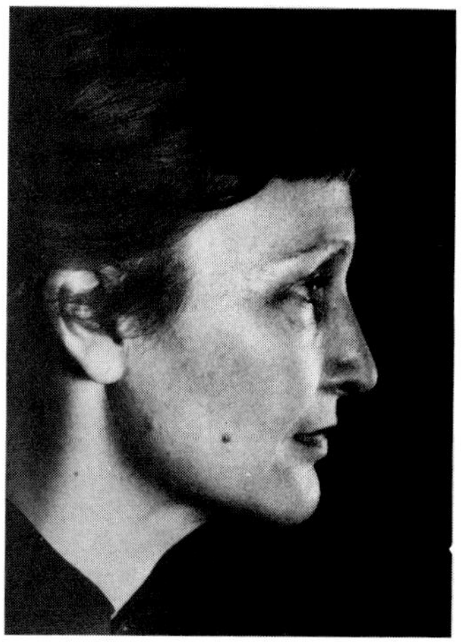

PHOTO 27: The preoperative sketch of planned rasping of her nasal hump and tip lift.

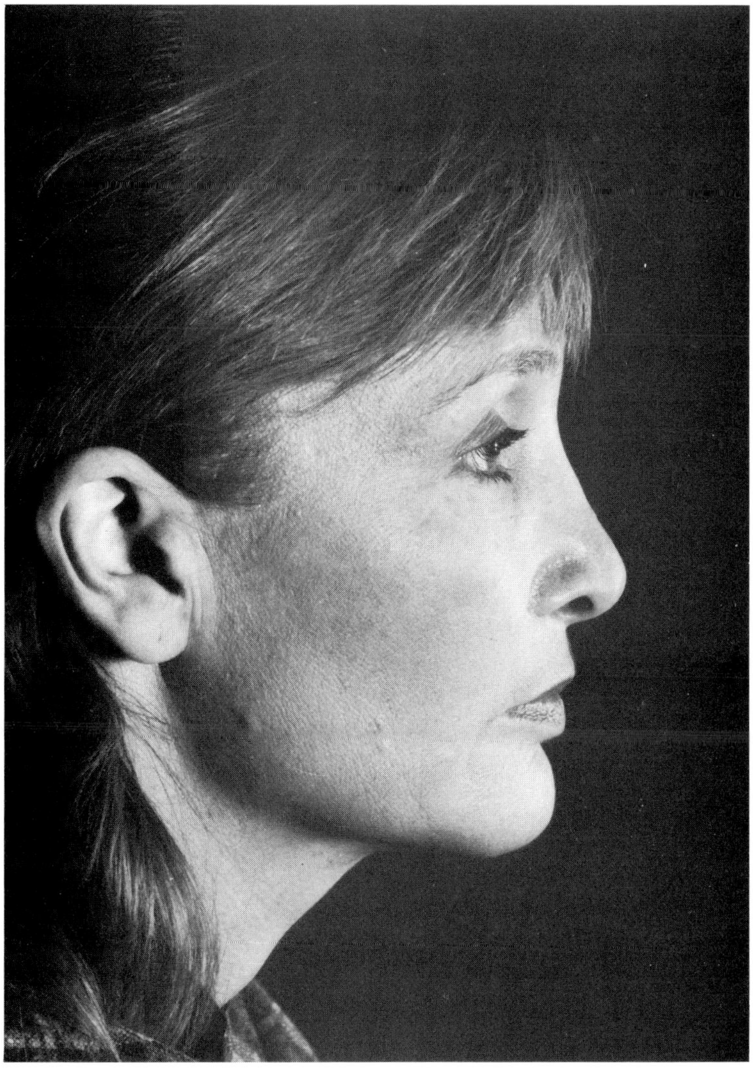

PHOTO 28: The same patient after *rhinoplasty*.

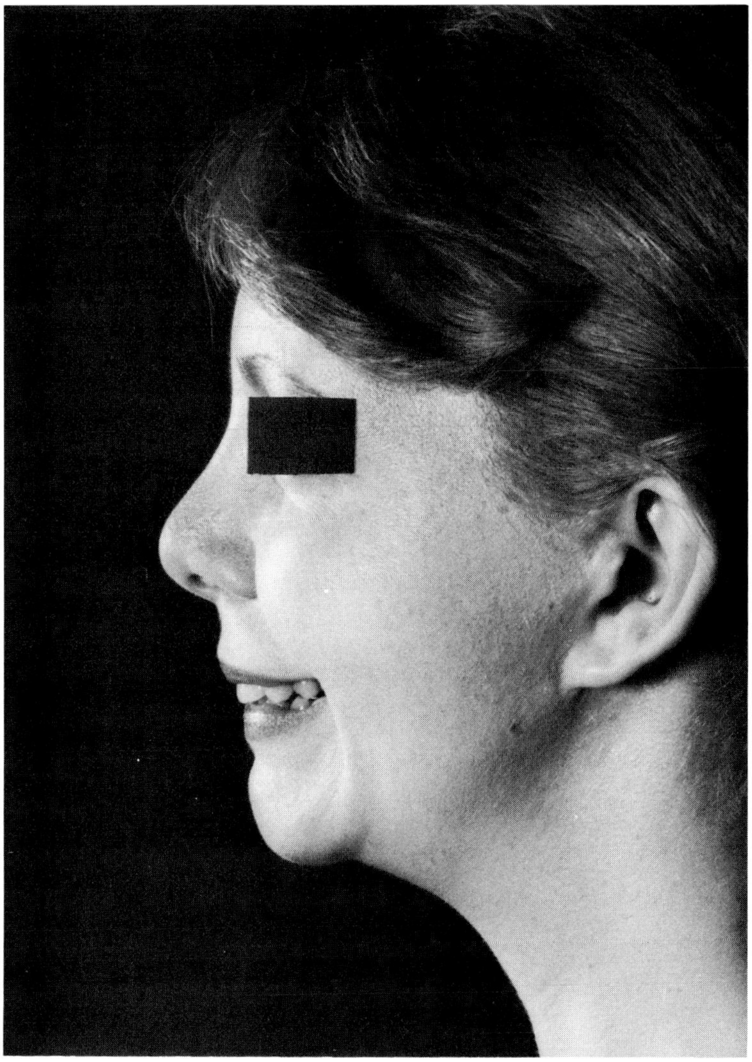

PHOTO 29: A patient with an ill-defined nasal tip after *primary rhinoplasty* elsewhere.

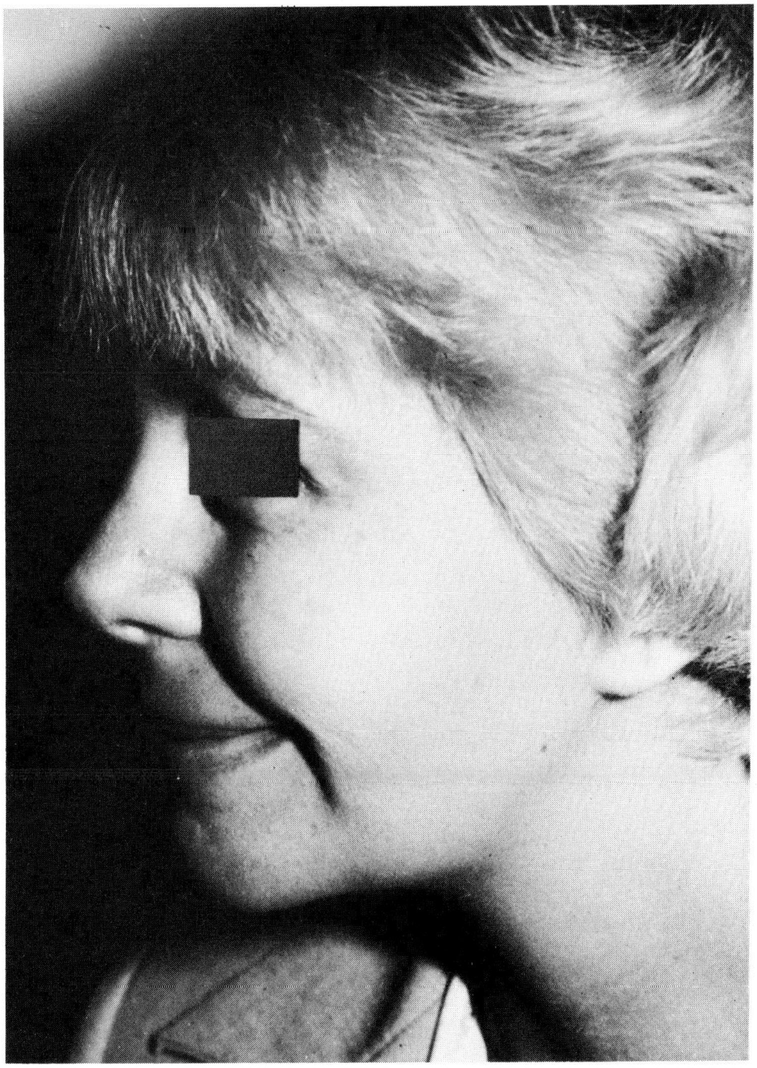

PHOTO 30: The same patient after *secondary rhinoplasty* to improve tip definition.

FINISHING TOUCHES

About 10–15% of patients undergoing *reduction rhinoplasty* would benefit as well from augmentation of the chin. Segments of the face should relate to the whole in a harmonious relationship as they do in all those celebrated beautiful faces of paintings, statues and individuals. In the case of a too small chin *(microgenia)* with normal *occlusion* or bite, a silicon implant may be inserted through an incision in the mouth to augment the chin. Skin tapes are allowed to remain in position on the chin until the nasal splint is removed. Thus convalescence is not prolonged and the surgical results can be greatly enhanced in appropriate patients by such *augmentation mentoplasty* (see **Photos 9–11**, **17–19** and **24–25**).

Since narrowing the nasal bridge makes the eyes appear wider, this effect can be augmented by removing any redundant skin or bags from the eyelids with *blepharoplasty* to complete the "brighter-eyed" picture (see **Photos 7** and **8**).

As discussed in the previous chapter, patients with flat faces or "dish-face" deformity can profit by *maxillary augmentation.* Placement of such implants through the intranasal incision can greatly improve facial proportion in those patients suffering from flat upper lips, upper lips less prominent than full lower lips, and deep hollows beneath and to the side of the nostrils.

It is not uncommon for many patients with broad noses to have not very prominent cheek bones. If the *cheek bone augmentation* is performed after the nose has been narrowed, the effect will be twice as dramatic and much greater than can be attained by either procedure alone. A face can be almost completely transformed.

CHAPTER 23

Prominent Ears Placed into Perspective

In Japan, large ears are considered a sign of good fortune. However, this is not true in Western culture, where large or prominent ears impose a stigma, causing the child with such ears to become an object of ridicule. The primary reason for operating on prominent ears is to eliminate this psychological trauma which the ear deformity can produce. Children can be extremely cruel, and the child with prominent ears is reminded frequently of this deformity by taunts from playmates. Females can conceal moderate degrees of ear deformity with hair styles, but if the ears are very prominent practically no hair style can conceal them.

Prominent ears stand out from the head by virtue of either a more obtuse angle between the ear and the side of the head or increased width of the cup portion, termed *conchal cartilage*, holding the ear from the side of the head (see **Fig. 16**). This condition may be unilateral or bilateral. 2 cm (3/4″) seems to be the upper limit of normal for the distance between the outside border of the ear *(superior helical rim)* and the head.

The ear is almost fully grown by the age of seven or eight years. By the time a child is three, the ear has achieved 85% of its growth potential although its growth in height continues into late adulthood. The ideal time for correction is thus the year before the child starts school. This prevents school playmates from inflicting psychic trauma upon the child and allows sufficient growth of the ear to have occurred.

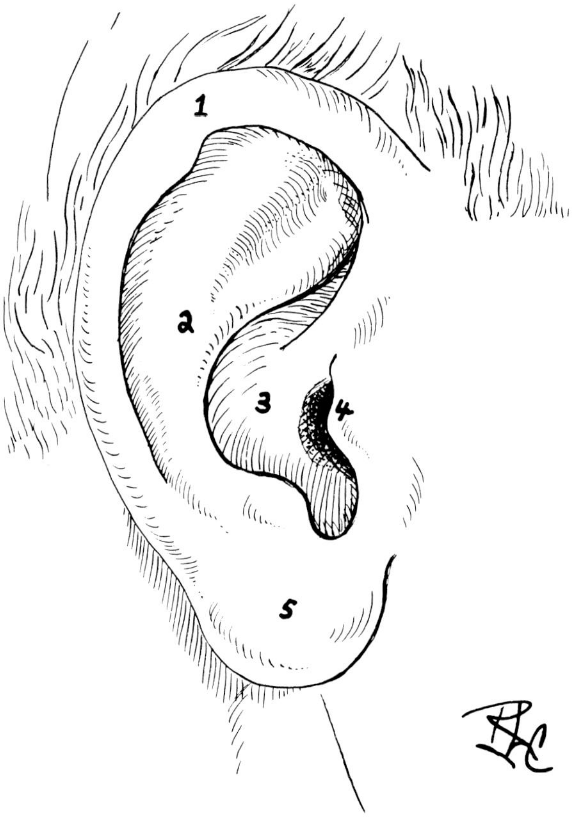

FIGURE 16: Anatomy of the normal ear: 1—*helical rim*; 2—*antihelical fold*; 3—*conchal cartilage*; 4—*tragus*; 5—earlobe. (Reprinted from *The Kindest Cut*.)

The usual deformity stems from the failure of folding of the inner convolutions of the ear *(antihelical fold)* between the third and sixth month *in utero.* The basic treatment consists of restoration of the inner convolutions of the ear and resection of extra *conchal cartilage* if necessary. The cartilage is scratched to allow it to bend backwards and it is fastened in that position with sutures. An ellipse of skin is similarly excised in back of the ear to help guarantee the maintenance of the ear in its modified position. The scar is located behind the ear and thus is not visible. For this surgery, young children usually require general anesthesia, but patients over 10 years of age do quite well under local, if properly sedated, unless extensive revision is anticipated.

After the surgery, a tightly molded dressing is placed to prevent bleeding and to allow healing in the proper position. It is usually kept intact for 3–4 days and is critically important to the finished result. After removal of this dressing, a stockinette headcap or other ear guard is usually worn at night for the first two weeks to protect the ears from twisting or bending with rupture of the internal sutures before healing is complete.

Few patients are born with ears perfectly equidistant from the side of the head, just as arms, legs, breasts or testes are not exactly the same size. The surgeon usually can do better than nature in this regard, but slight discrepancies occasionally occur. When they do, minor adjustments may be indicated and performed in the office.

CASE HISTORY

S.N. was a 26-year-old physical therapist who had never been able to wear her hair up because of prominent ears. She had always wanted to have this fixed but had put it off until a friend of hers underwent the procedure and said "it was nothing." She had been the object of the usual "Mickey Mouse" and "Dumbo" jokes in grade school.

Under local anesthesia in the office, the poorly-formed internal convolutions were restored so that her ears assumed their proper places. She was ecstatic with the result and wore her hair up for all postoperative visits to "show them off".

PREPARATION

Vitamin K and Vitamin C are prescribed and *aspirin-containing drugs and Vitamin E are avoided for two weeks preoperatively. Medical photo-*

graphs are taken. The hair is shampooed and the face washed with *Phisohex®* on the morning of surgery.

Most adults and older children prefer the office for the surgery which is performed under local anesthesia. It is generally best to put younger children in the hospital for general anesthesia.

THE PROCEDURE

After preliminary sedation and intravenous relaxants, the skin behind and in front of the ear is numbed with local anesthetic. Through a short incision on the back of the ear, a specially-made instrument is tunneled beneath the skin, over the rim of the ear, onto the front surface of the cartilage, and used to score it at the site of proper bending *(antihelical fold)*.

The ear will then bend into its proper location unless there is also extra cartilage present *(concha)*. If this is the case, as it is in about one-quarter of patients, a small portion of this redundant cartilage is removed. The edges of its removal are suitably beveled to give a natural front contour.

Stitches are then inserted on the back surface to maintain the convolutions and projection of the ear in the desired position. The incision on the back of the ear is then closed with a continuous stitch.

Cotton dipped in mineral oil is used to make a molded turban dressing which conforms exactly to the ear. This dressing is allowed to remain in place for at least 3 days. A scarf or cap can be used to cover it when the patient leaves the office.

RECUPERATION

The dressing is generally removed on the 3rd or 4th day. The patient may be seen socially at this time. The front of the ear may be slightly discolored for a week or two but usually this is not very noticeable. The stitches are removed on the 10th day.

I recommend that patients wear a stockinette head cap or ear band at night for the first two weeks to prevent the ears from accidently bending during sleep. Normal athletics such as jogging or tennis may be resumed at two weeks but I recommend that contact sports be avoided for an additional week. A typical result is illustrated in **Photos 31** and **32**.

PRECAUTIONS AND POTENTIAL PROBLEMS

As in all surgery, bleeding rarely may occur and cause a collection of blood termed a *hematoma.* The molded cotton dressing is designed specifically to prevent this. Such a collection would be evacuated and the turban dressing be replaced for a few days.

Asymmetry in projection of the two ears may rarely occur. It is correctible by a minor office adjustment. Good surgery results in more symmetry than nature which accepts an average of 1° greater projection of the right ear than the left.

Infection occurs very rarely and would be managed by appropriate antibiotics. It is possible for the surgeon to be forced to remove the internal sutures although I have never encountered this situation. Since the cartilage has been scored for bending, correction would still be maintained.

* * *

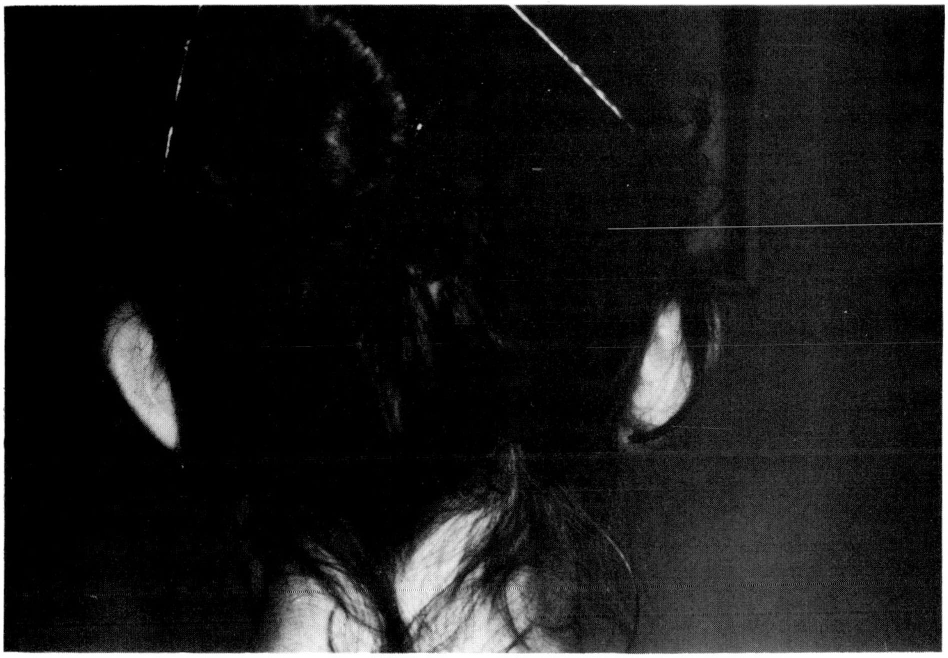

PHOTO 31:.A back view of a woman with prominent ears.

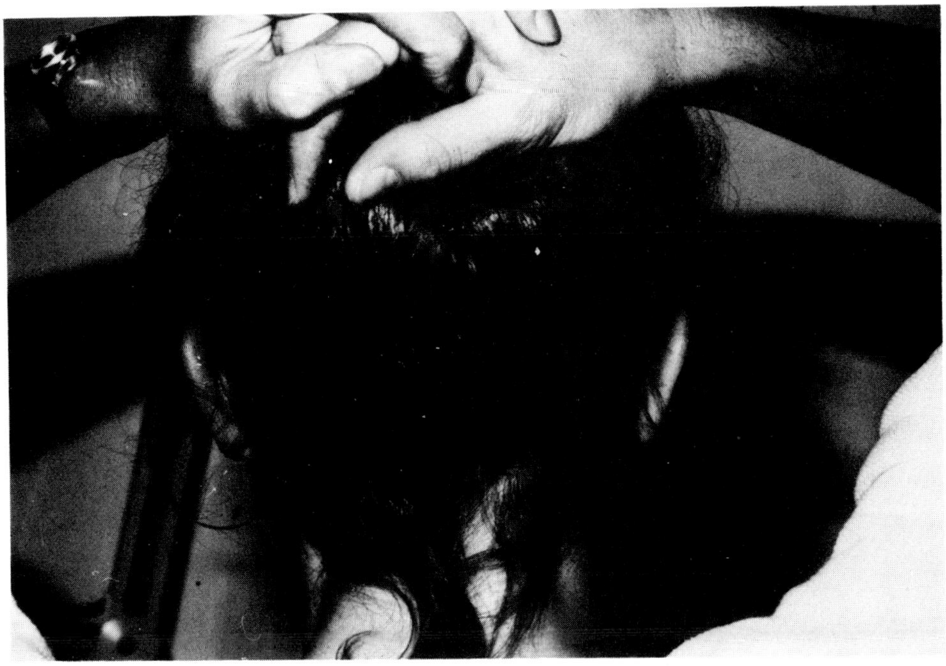

PHOTO 32: The same patient after *otoplasty*.

FINISHING TOUCHES

Most ladies change their hairstyles postoperatively in favor of the more sophisticated styles that prominent ears have prevented them from wearing. *Large earlobes may be reduced* at the time of ear surgery and *earlobes may be pierced* if this is desired since many female patients start wearing earrings for the first time postoperatively.

Since patients undergoing ear surgery generally comprise a young population, the most frequent, associated procedure in my practice is *rhinoplasty* to refine a bulbous nasal tip.

* * *

Afterword—
Facing the Future

As we have discussed the "state of the art" of plastic surgery, we have seen how to *preserve what Nature has given us for the longest possible time and in the best possible condition.* We have also seen how *some of Nature's mistakes can be corrected* and how *some of our own indiscretions can be remedied* after-the-fact. We have even seen how *the normal aging process can be somewhat slowed through preventative skin care* and *the clock can be turned back through surgery.*

DMSO appeared to be the ideal vehicle for bringing substances across the skin. Hopes were raised that it could carry moisturizers to the dermis, anti-arthritis drugs into the joints, and have a multitude of other uses. Unfortunately, it is not devoid of side effects, such as causing cataracts! No doubt, more ideal vehicles will be discovered which can carry moisturizers and nutrients deeper into the skin and help us further to care for the skin.

What about the frontiers in the field of plastic surgery? What will the next decade hold for us? I feel the *Argon LASER* will probably become the method of choice for the treatment of spiders *(telangiectasias)* and the vascular tumors *(hemangiomas)* that affect 10% of children. If LASERS are refined to the point of being able to damage fewer cells than the blade of a scalpel, then the *CO_2 LASER* may surplant the surgical scalpel as well.

Plastic surgery will always have use for an injectable soft tissue filler. While currently available collagen preparations are useful for many applications, they are not suitable for deeper or bulk augmentation. I believe that we will create an injectable biologic extract that "cross-links" in the body after injection and has a very small amount of absorption. *Elastin* may well be the source of this compound.

Newer *dissociative drugs* will be developed, akin to *ketamine* which has several drawbacks, that allow an even greater scope of surgical procedures to be performed safely and comfortably under local anaesthesia in the office. Office surgery will become more and more common as surgeons add efficient Operating Rooms to their offices. Financial considerations, insurance companies, scheduling considerations, and probably eventually the government will force this transition.

As the more extensive procedures become safe enough for cosmetic applications, I believe that the principles of *craniofacial surgery* (repositioning the bones of the face and skull) which have developed out of the treatment of severe congenital defects, will be more commonly applied to solely cosmetic alterations of the facial bone structure.

Microsurgery will become more and more pervasive in the transplantation of lost parts and it will become common to move tissue from one part of the body to another electively for cosmetic purposes as well as reconstructive ones.

Biologically benign *tissue glues* may eventually replace sutures and *synthetic blood substitutes* will make the fear of blood loss a thing of the past. As *cell cultures* and *tissue banks* get more sophisticated, it will be possible to take a small sample of a specific tissue, grow more of it, and use it when the need arises. For example, it will be possible to take a small piece of skin, and then grow out sheets of skin to use in a severe burn—the patient's own skin! Great strides are being made in this direction right now. Perhaps cells in the tissue culture can be made to develop by nuclear manipulation into complex tissues and even whole organs!

Computers have revolutionized inventory, invoicing and secretarial tasks. As microchips are being developed with larger and larger capacities, smaller and more versatile units appear with new applications. The Computer Transaxial Tomogram *(CTT)* has revolutionized radiologic diagnosis; I believe we will see the computer's eventual application to treatment as well with "processing" of special scans for particular purposes. The patient will be scanned, the computer will process the scan along pre-programmed guidelines for "aesthetic ideals", and then display the potential results of lifting procedures, profiloplasties, craniofacial surgeries, and soft tissue augmentations—most likely, *holographically*, in three dimensions! Fortunately, plastic surgeons will still have to perform the surgery. However, I could envision computerized correction of soft tissue defects with injectable fillers!

As far-fetched as the above scenario may sound, it is not as exciting as the concept of *genetic engineering.* Our cells are pre-programmed to become obsolescent and die. Cancer may indeed be an aging phenomenon! If we could "turn off" this aging process, all of the lifting procedures would be a thing of the past. Congenital defects and undersireable family traits could be averted by genetic alterations in the womb. Genetic pre-programming for such traits as male-pattern baldness could be eliminated. Surgical treatment of cancer might be passe! Plastic surgeons might only need be around to repair the results of trauma. But this need would only be present until we learned to program our bodies to respond to the loss of parts by regeneration as do several "lower life forms".

Sounds Exciting? Yes, but the implications are also a little frightening at the same time! We may not have lived up to all the expectations of the 60's, but we have made great strides in the last decade. I feel medicine and surgery will make important advances in the next and subsequent decades; and plastic surgery, as one of the most pioneering and consumer-oriented subspecialties, will be in the forefront in applying these new technologies.

* * *